It All Begins With The Egg:

How the Science of Egg Quality Can Increase Your Chances of Getting Pregnant, Avoid Miscarriage, And Help You Conceive Naturally

BY

TERESA J. MACEK

COPYRIGHT

Disclaimer

The information provided in this book is for general informational purposes only. It is not intended to be a substitute for professional advice. The author and publisher make no representation or warranties of any kind regarding the completeness, accuracy, reliability, suitability, or availability of the information contained herein.

ABOUT THE AUTHOR PAGE

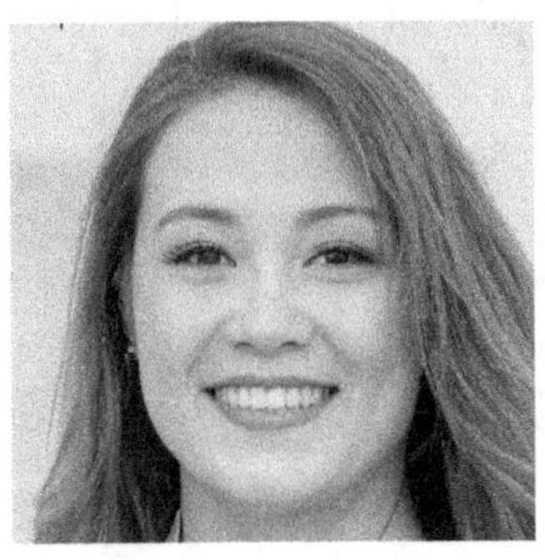

The perceptive author of "It All Begins With The Egg," Teresa J. Macek, is a specialist in the science of reproduction and a fervent supporter of reproductive health. Teresa, has devoted her professional life to elucidating the intricacies of reproductive science and enabling people to make the most of their own paths to parenting.

Teresa aims to demystify the world of reproductive health in a way that is both approachable and empowering by combining a deep awareness of scientific nuances with a caring approach to the human experience, served as the inspiration for her journey into the field of fertility, and this intimate connection lends realism and relatability to each page of the book.

Teresa provides a plethora of information in "It All Begins With The Egg," which she has amassed over years of study, research, and real-world experience. The book functions as a thorough guide, giving readers an understanding of the science behind egg quality and practical suggestions for boosting natural fertility, increasing the likelihood of conception, and preventing miscarriages.

Teresa is a strong proponent of closing the knowledge gap between science and practical application because she understands that information is an incredibly useful tool for anyone pursuing parenthood. Every chapter in "It All Begins With The Egg" demonstrates her commitment to giving people and couples a road map for navigating the complex process of fertility with resiliency, hope, and informed decision-making.

Allow Teresa J. Macek to be your guide as you set out on this fascinating trip through the science of fertility. She offers not only her expertise but also a supportive hand and voice.

Teresa has written profound books on parenting and family. To get to see all of Teresa's books, scan the barcode.

TABLE OF CONTENT

It All Begins With The Egg:

INTRODUCTION

Welcome to the unusual world of reproductive science, where eggs take center stage and the drama is more riveting than your favorite reality TV program! I'm Teresa J. Macek, and I'll be your trusted guide through the journey of conception, miscarriage prevention, and natural conception. Buckle up, because we're about to embark on a journey that combines science, wit, and my personal fertility rodeo experiences.

Consider this: a frantic lady (myself), armed with a salad spinner, a yoga mat, and enough fertility apps to make a tech guru blush. Yes, I was on a quest to solve the egg quality code. I had no idea that my pursuit of the perfect poached egg would lead to an obsession with reproductive health science.

Now, let me take you back to the day I realized my ovaries had a "best by" date. Spoiler alert: it is not printed on the package. As I peered down the barrel of my biological clock, I wondered, "If only there was a user manual for these ovaries!" That is how the concept for this book was born (no pun intended).

"It All Begins With The Egg" isn't your normal fertility handbook; rather, it's a behind-the-scenes look into your reproductive system. We'll look at how egg quality may make or shatter your reproductive aspirations, and I'll try my best to keep it as interesting as a Netflix marathon.

As we get into the nitty-gritty of reproductive science, I'll weave in anecdotes that will make you laugh, cringe, and possibly shed a tear or two. After all, what's life without a sense of humor, especially while dealing with hormones and fertility treatments?

So, whether you're looking for a good chuckle, some sound counsel, or just to figure out what I did with that salad spinner, "It All Begins With The Egg" is your backstage pass to fertility, served with a side of fun and a dollop of science.

Let the eggstravaganza begin! 🔍🎉.

It All Begins With The Egg:

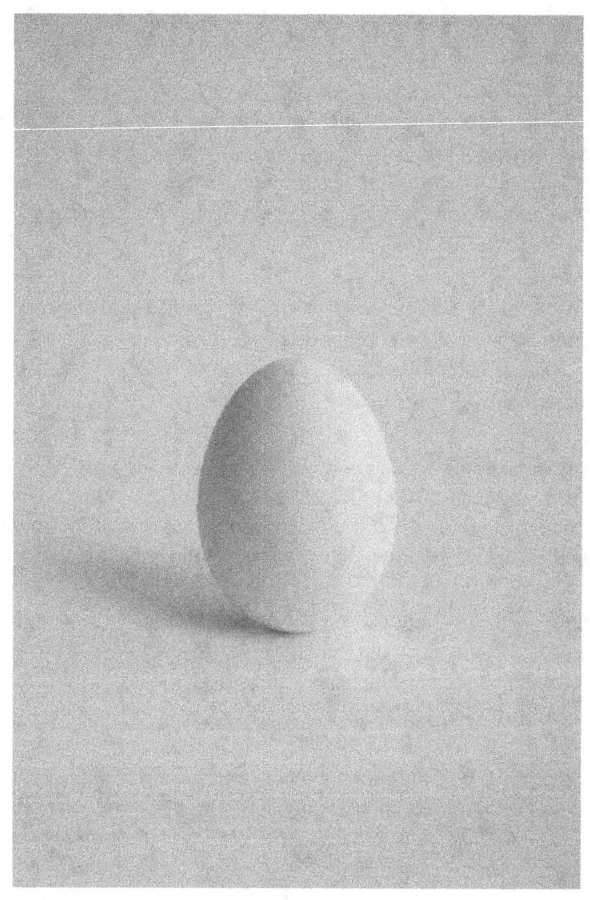

Chapter 1
The Egg and Its Significance

Chapter 1

The Egg and Its Significance

The most amazing human cell is an egg, which, when triggered, can develop into a fully formed person in a few days or weeks. In any higher animal, no other cell possesses this ability. The union of an egg and sperm during fertilization is typically the result of activation. However, in some animals, an egg can be artificially activated by a number of nonspecific chemical or physical treatments, and the sperm itself is not strictly necessary. In fact, parthenogenetically—the reproduction of certain organisms, including a few vertebrates like lizards—some species typically reproduce from eggs that become activated in the absence of sperm.

Even though an egg can develop into any sort of cell in an adult body, it is a highly specialized cell that is only able to perform the singular task of creating a new individual. Even the nucleus of a somatic cell can be reprogrammed by the cytoplasm of an egg to control the formation of a new person.Naturally, women's ovaries are designed to only enable one egg to develop, mature, and release (also known as "ovulating") throughout each cycle, which typically occurs once a month. The single egg signifies the solitary opportunity for conception during that specific menstrual cycle.

It's possible that the ovulated egg was aberrant or normal. If everything is normal, congratulations! Your pregnancy is healthy. However, what if it isn't? When abnormal egg cells fertilize or implant in the uterus, they usually do not cause miscarriage or genetic diseases such as Down syndrome. However, in rare instances, they may cause these problems.

The statistical probability that the one egg a woman has ovulated is normal determines the difference in egg quality between a 25-year-old and a 40-year-old. It's much more likely that the one egg a woman produces each month will be abnormal because women in their late 30s and early 40s have a larger percentage of abnormal eggs. This explains why age-related losses in natural fertility occur, and why women over 35 are more likely to have infertility, miscarriage, and genetic abnormalities.

Anatomy Of Egg

What Is A Human Egg Cell

The main reproductive organs that create gametes are gonads. In males, two testes yield sperm, and in females, two ovaries yield ovum. An ovum, also known as an egg cell, is a female reproductive cell that unites with sperm during fertilization. This ovum goes through a process known as oogenesis to become its mature form.

This ovum is fertilized inside the female's body in viviparous mammals. In contrast, the uterus is where the embryo develops.

Structure Of The Ovum

One of the biggest cells is the ovum, which has a diameter of about 120 μm. The ovum contains a large, cytoplasm-covered nucleus positioned in the center. The terms "germinal vesicle" and "germinal disc" refer to the nucleolus and nucleus of this egg, respectively. Similarly, ooplasm refers to the cytoplasm (yolk) of an ovum. Because it contains less yolk than a person would, it is alecithal. The cortex, a peripheral layer with many microvilli, encloses this ooplasm. The plasmalemma's tubular projections, known as microvilli, help move materials into and out of the cytoplasm.

Normally, the human ovum has three layers covering it:

- → thin vitelline membrane within
- → intermediate pellucid zone
- → outer radiating corona

The perivitelline space is the thin area that exists between the zona pellucida and the vitelline membrane. The corona radiata encircles the zona pellucida, which is frequently perceived as a thick girdle.

The center zona pellucida of an ovulated egg must be separated from the outer corona radiata by the sperm acrosome's hyaluronidase in order for fertilization to take place. This always permits contact between the sperm and the core of the oocyte.

Functions Of Embryogenesis

The ovum is essential to the process of fertilization, as was previously established. The ovum enters the fallopian tube through the fimbriated end during ovulation. The cilia on the inner side of the fimbriated end shift to allow the ovum to enter. Ovulation is the process by which an adult follicle releases its ovum. It is found in the ovary at the primary oocyte stage, when it has 23 pairs of diploid chromosomes. Just prior to ovulation, the ovum goes through the meiotic division process. Thus, the original oocyte divides into a secondary oocyte and a first polar body. Following the expulsion of the first polar body, the secondary oocyte—which is haploid and only has 23 chromosomes—remains. The first polar body is ejected together with the remaining 23 chromosomes.

The female gamete, which is in its secondary oocyte stage, cleaves into a second polar body and a mature ovum shortly after fertilization. Subsequently, the second polar body is released as well. The developed ovum's nucleus now develops into a female pronucleus with 22 autosomes and one sex chromosome (X).

Role Of Egg Quality In Successful Conception

QUALITY OF EGG

A woman's capacity to become fertile and produce a child is significantly influenced by the quality of her eggs. The best chance for an embryo to develop, implant in the uterus, and produce a healthy pregnancy is with high-quality eggs.

Whether an egg is chromosomally "normal" (euploid) or "abnormal" (aneuploid) is referred to as its quality. A chromosomally normal egg contains 23 chromosomes, and the subsequent chromosomally normal embryo will have 46 chromosomes overall after fertilization by the sperm, which likewise contains 23 chromosomes.

EGG QUALITY AND AGE

An increasing number of aneuploid eggs—eggs with either too few or too many chromosomes—are produced by an aging ovary in a woman. Aneuploid eggs will result in an embryo with either too few or too many chromosomes if conception takes place. The majority of aneuploid embryos either miscarry or fail to implant in the uterus. An additional copy of chromosome 21 or chromosomal abnormalities like Down syndrome can occasionally be caused by aneuploid embryos.

Seventy percent of a woman's eggs have normal chromosomes at thirty years of age. About 60% of a woman's eggs are chromosomally normal at 35 years old. About 35 percent of a woman's eggs are chromosomally normal by the time she is 40.

QUANTITY OF EGG

A woman has between one and two million eggs at birth, which is her entire egg supply. At various phases of development, the ovaries contain eggs in the form of follicles, which gradually decrease in quantity and quality. Her ovarian reserve will contain about 300,000 potential eggs by the time she enters puberty. She will only ovulate a few hundred eggs in her reproductive years.

Our fertility specialists can determine how well you will respond to ovarian-stimulating medications based on your age, medical history, and the findings of your ovarian reserve testing (see below). We can also create a customized care plan for your specific needs related to reproductive treatment. Recall that all it takes to develop an embryo is one healthy egg and one sperm!

Testing of Ovarians Reserve

We can assess your overall reproductive potential and establish whether you are ovulating with the following blood tests and ultrasound.

i) Tests For Hormones That Stimulates Follicles (Fsh)

We can draw blood on the third day of the menstrual cycle in order to measure the hormone FSH, which is essential for the growth of new follicles. The pituitary gland in the brain communicates with the ovaries through FSH. Every month, it tells the ovaries when it's time to produce an egg. It requires more and more FSH to maintain the cycle when the quality of the eggs declines because they become less sensitive to the hormone. Consequently, the quality of the eggs decreases with increasing FSH levels.

ii) Estradiol (E2)

The ovaries' way of talking to the brain is through the hormone E2, which is the companion of FSH. When an ovarian follicle grows larger and gets more stimulated, E2 levels rise. The estradiol level should be less than 50 pg/ml in order to be evaluated and to guarantee the validity of the FSH value. Early in the cycle, if it is higher than 50 pg/ml, the ovaries are responding early and the quality of the eggs may be compromised.

iii) Amh, Or Anti-Mullerian Hormone

The granulosa cells of early developing eggs secrete a glycoprotein called AMH, which aids in the protection and maturation of the eggs. Over the course of a lifetime, AMH and granulosa cells diminish in tandem with a decline in the number of eggs. The amount of eggs that are still in the ovary is estimated by AMH.

iv) Transvaginal Sonography

We are able to determine the resting/antral follicle count (AFC) via a transvaginal ultrasound. The ultrasound is often done between days three and twelve of your menstrual cycle. It counts all of the follicles in both ovaries that measure between four and nine millimeters. These are potentially developed eggs that will eventually be ovulated. If you have fewer follicles, you can experience issues with the amount and quality of your eggs.

FREEZING EGG

Oocyte vitrification, oocyte cryopreservation, and/or fertility preservation are other names for egg freezing, which allows women who aren't ready to have children now but would like to in the future. The mature eggs inside the ovaries are removed, frozen, and kept until you decide to use them after taking ovarian stimulating medicine.

You have a better chance of becoming pregnant later in life if you freeze your eggs when they are more abundant and of higher quality.

Egg Quality And Fertility Are Indirectly Related.
Naturally, women's ovaries are designed to only enable one egg to develop, mature, and release (also known as "ovulating") throughout each cycle, which typically occurs once a month. The single egg signifies the solitary opportunity for conception during that specific menstrual cycle.

It's possible that the ovulated egg was aberrant or normal. If everything is normal, congratulations! Your pregnancy is healthy. However, what if it isn't? When abnormal egg cells fertilize or implant in the uterus, they usually do not cause miscarriage or genetic diseases such as Down syndrome. However, in rare instances, they may cause these problems.

The statistical probability that the one egg a woman has ovulated is normal determines the difference in egg quality between a 25-year-old and a 40-year-old. It's much more likely that the one egg a woman produces each month will be abnormal because women in their late 30s and early 40s have a larger percentage of abnormal eggs. This explains why age-related losses in natural fertility occur, and why women over 35 are more likely to have infertility, miscarriage, and genetic abnormalities.

Your Chance At Pregnancy Is Derived By The Age Of The Egg.
Research has shown that women who use their own eggs that are the same age for in vitro fertilization have far lower success rates (see chart below). Nonetheless, the 51% pregnancy rate for those who used donor eggs from a younger woman remained consistent across all age categories.

This supported a crucial finding: the age of the egg has the greatest bearing on fertility since it directly connects to egg quality and, consequently, to the egg's capacity to fertilize into a healthy pregnancy. A youthful, healthy egg usually results in a healthy pregnancy, but there are certain hazards involved with having a pregnancy at what is known as "advanced maternal age," including a slightly higher risk of gestational diabetes and preeclampsia.

It All Begins With The Egg:

Egg freezing is effective because it enables women to preserve the quality of their young, healthy eggs and freeze them, enabling them to become their own egg donors in the future.

How to Improve the Quality of Your Eggs While Trying to Get Pregnant

Ladies, the biological clock is a real thing, and as such, getting older lowers your chances of getting pregnant and raises the possibility that you will miscarry. This is due to the fact that by the time you are 40, fewer than half of your eggs are regarded as "normal," which primarily affects your ovarian environment and your chances of becoming pregnant. The good news is that by implementing a few healthy lifestyle adjustments, you can improve your ovarian environment.

Actions You Can Take

Your chromosomally normal or defective egg quality is mostly determined by your biological family tree in addition to your age. This may result in a successful pregnancy or infertility. Unfortunately, your egg quality declines as you get older, making ovulation and fertilization more difficult in your latter 30s and early 40s. Therefore, if you are attempting to conceive (TTC), you should be aware that optimal odds for conception can be achieved by improving the quality of your eggs, because doing so will provide a solid basis for a fruitful pregnancy.

1) Managing Stress To Your Advantage: When you're under stress, your body releases hormones like prolactin and cortisol that disrupt the development of eggs. Walking, yoga, and meditation are all excellent methods to reduce unhealthy stress levels. Warm baths are also a great way to de-stress. They also help to normalize your immune system and improve blood flow to your reproductive organs.

2) Eat A Balanced Diet: Eating meals high in nutrients improves the quality and health of eggs. To provide your body the nourishment it needs to sustain your eggs, include whole grains, lean meats, leafy greens, fresh vegetables, fruit, and nuts in your diet. Steer clear of processed foods and meats whenever you can, and consume less sugar and salt.

3) Retain A Healthy Weight: A healthy body mass index, or BMI, is what you should aim for. Being overweight reduces both the quantity and quality of your eggs. Your hormone balance is impacted by obesity, which may prevent ovulation. By balancing your reproductive hormones and reducing inflammation, which otherwise limits blood supply to the ovaries, a high-fat, low-carb diet enhances overall fertility and egg quality. Additionally, fat supports cell growth and provides your body with the energy it needs to conceive.

4) Add Omega3 To Your Diet: You may want to take fish oil (Omega 3s), melatonin, and coenzyme Q10. Antioxidants from these supplements increase ovarian function, improve egg quality, and improve sleep quality. Omega 3 fatty acids maintain fecundity and improve the quality of eggs, and Q10 offers antioxidant protection for your mitochondria. This provides your body with the energy it needs to replicate DNA and produce more high-quality eggs. While taking vitamin E reduces oxidative stress and increases follicular blood supply—which is required for high-quality eggs—taking vitamin A enhances oocyte quality and embryo development. B vitamins also support the production of DNA. Consuming zinc has been shown to support the production of high-quality oocytes, and supplementing with folate improves oocyte maturation, fertilization, and implantation.

5) Get A Good Night's Sleep: Fertility and egg quality are closely correlated with sleep. It enables your body to produce hormones like melatonin, repair damaged cells, and replenish energy. Melatonin promotes oocyte quality, ovulation, and embryo development, all of which are essential to reproductive processes and the production of healthy, high-quality eggs in your body. This is particularly beneficial because women's melatonin levels decrease beyond the age of forty.

6) Improve Blood Flow: Healthy eggs are produced when the body receives oxygen-rich blood. It's an excellent idea to drink 64 ounces of water a day to prevent dehydration! Moreover, yoga poses including the lotus, child, and reclining hero might increase blood flow.

7) Avoid Cigarettes: The toxins in cigarettes speed up the loss of eggs from your ovaries and alter the DNA of your egg cells, making them unusable for pregnancy.

It All Begins With The Egg:

8) Avoid Alcohol And Caffeine: These two substances disrupt the processes involved in conception; therefore, to enhance the quality of your eggs, cut back on your alcohol intake.

9) Freeze Your Eggs Right Away: As the quality of your eggs deteriorates with age, this is done to guarantee the best quality and chances of conception. To combat that, freeze your eggs now using cryopreservation, ensuring that they maintain their freshness and health from the day they were frozen!

Improving Egg Quality Techniques

You can adhere to the following tactics in order to improve the quality of your eggs and start your parenthood as soon as possible.

A. Nutritional Supplements

A variety of nutritional supplements can be used to prepare the body for conception, depending on the particular needs of the pair.

i) Folic Acid

This B vitamin significantly improves the chances of conception. Furthermore, folic acid aids in the prevention of congenital spinal and brain abnormalities.

Natural Folic Acid Sources:
- Whole Grains
- Legumes and green, leafy vegetables.
- Fatty Acids Omega-3
- Healthy fats called omega-3 fatty acids assist in balancing the hormones involved in reproduction. In addition, these fats support the regulation of implantation and menstruation.

Natural Sources Of Omega-3
- Fish oil,
- algae oil
- tuna or sardines
- salmon.

ii) CoQ10

CoQ10 is a potent antioxidant found in nature that enhances ovarian responsiveness. Moreover, it shields the eggs from oxidative harm.

Natural Sources Of Coenzyme Q10-.
- ➔ Fish
- ➔ Meat

B) Refrain From Self-Medication Since It Could Have Unfavorable Effects.
I sincerely hope that you would always seek the advice of a reproductive specialist prior to using dietary supplements to increase fertility.

C) Mind-Body Practices:
A deeper level of self-awareness and mindfulness can be attained by comprehending the relationship between the mind and body. It assists in adjusting to the changes that occur both before and during pregnancy. Massage therapy, meditation, yoga, deep breathing exercises, and general bodily relaxation are among the best mind-body therapies.

D) Fertility Treatments
Since its introduction, Assisted Reproductive Technology (ART) has brought millions of infertile couples around the world closer to becoming parents. Depending on their problems and medical conditions, infertile individuals have a wide range of the following possibilities.

i) IVF: During this medical technique, the eggs are removed and placed on a petri dish so that their quality may be examined. After fertilization, the high-quality eggs are placed inside the uterus.
ii) Intracytoplasmic Sperm Injection (Icsi): Involves injecting the sperm directly into the egg. The quantity of fertilized eggs can be boosted with the aid of ICSI. It can only be carried out if there are no infertility problems with the male partner.

Nutritious Assistance For High-Quality Eggs

It is impossible to overstate the importance of diet on fertility. Your pregnancy dream may come true or not depending on what you put into your body.

Superfoods and Antioxidants: Eating a diet rich in dietary antioxidants and fertility superfoods can improve the quality of eggs.

The Following Are The Best Superfoods To Maintain Egg Quality:
→ Asparagus
→ Lentils with beans
→ Sprouts
→ yolks of eggs
→ Cashews
→ Sweet potatoes
→ Berries

Do you want to know which antioxidants are greatest for fertility? Eat that fruit, then!

Fruits Rich In Antioxidants Include:
→ Apples
→ Oranges
→ Pomegranates
→ Grapes
→ Kiwis
→ Grapefruit.

B. Anti-Inflammatory Diet: Although the term may imply an ostentatious diet, it's not! Every fruit and vegetable has anti-inflammatory qualities.

You can create a vibrant bowl of grains, fruits, veggies, healthy fats, and other ingredients to start your anti-inflammatory diet. What you can do is as follows:

→ vegetables such as broccoli, cauliflower, cabbage, onions, radish, spinach, carrots, and garlic (which is high in selenium).

It All Begins With The Egg:

→ Make friends with berries; blackberries, raspberries, strawberries, and blueberries, among others.

→ Enjoy a tropical fruit such as a mango, pineapple, or banana.

→ Oranges and grapefruits, among other citrus fruits, are excellent.

→ Nuts and seeds such as sunflower, pumpkin, walnut, and chestnut seeds, as well as dates.

→ Barley, wheat, oats, whole rye, brown rice, and millet are examples of whole grains.

→ Rich sources of good fats include cold-pressed olive oil, avocados, and coconut oil.

→ Remember to have plenty of glasses of water!

The body becomes inflamed when it consumes foods heavy in sugar, saturated fats, junk food, and high processing levels. A hormone called cortisol is released by the body and it inhibits fertility. Thus, to preserve the quality of your eggs and increase your chances of becoming pregnant, make sure you stay away from such items.

Well-Being to Enhance Egg Quality

A sound body is supported by a sound mind. Read this line again! A calm mind will facilitate the benefits of all the vitamins you are taking, the healthy diet you are eating, and the treatment you are receiving to function more effectively.

Stress Management: One of the main obstacles to ovulation is stress. Prolactin and cortisol can be produced in excess while under stress. These stress hormones cause the ovaries to produce fewer eggs, which interferes with ovulation and fertilization. Consequently, managing mental stress becomes essential.

The greatest techniques to manage your stress include journaling, yoga, breathing techniques, meditation, and music listening.

Among the yoga poses that help with stress management and conception are
→ Surya Namaskar

→ Shodhan Nadi Yamada

→ Janu Shirasana

→ Baddha The Konasana

→ Bhramari Yamada

→ Balasana

→ Paschimottanasana

In addition to addressing mental and emotional exhaustion, regular practice of these asanas stimulates the ovaries. The flow of blood to the pelvic area has increased. These reproductive asanas also help your body get ready for a happy, healthy pregnancy.

The Benefits of Exercise and Sleep: It has been demonstrated that sleep is the finest medication. While you sleep, your body repairs itself trillions of times. With the appropriate exercises, this medication has the potential to significantly improve your journey. You can combine daily activities including walking, swimming, pilates, strength training, and fertility yoga asanas.

These will support a healthy BMI, reduce stress, and promote restful sleep. It's likely that being obese will negatively impact your fertility in some way.

Myths Regarding the Quality of Eggs
There are still a lot of false beliefs about fertility and egg quality. The idea that birth control drugs negatively impact egg quality is a prevalent one. According to experts, this is untrue. In actuality, birth control drugs occasionally aid to reduce the endometriosis's progression. It can therefore aid in reproduction.

It All Begins With The Egg:

It's also a common misconception that PCOS, a hormonal disorder characterized by enlarged ovaries, makes it impossible to conceive. It doesn't.

"It is important for those with PCOS, [which] affects 15% of women, to know about their condition and how to treat it from an early age—not just when they are ready to get pregnant," explains Dr. Eyvazzadeh.

The idea that egg quality may be specifically altered is a least common misconception. This is untrue for two key reasons.

Age and genetics have a direct influence on egg quality and cannot be changed or managed, claims Dr. Eyvazzadeh."

Mother Nature's impacts are unavoidable. However, you may try your best to understand and support the quality of your eggs by making informed decisions and taking appropriate action.

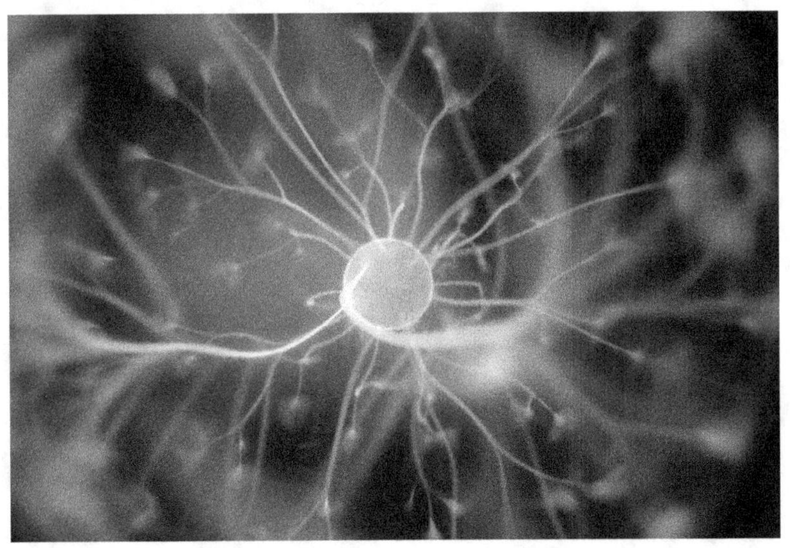

Chapter 2
The Start-Up Science

Chapter 2

The Start-Up Science

Exploring The Latest Scientific Advancements In Fertility

The lives of infertile couples, particularly women, are significantly impacted negatively by society by infertility; these individuals often endure emotional stress, sadness, anxiety, divorce, violence, and low self-esteem.

On the other hand, as technology develops daily, our lives continue to benefit from the gradual but significant changes.

Regarding fertility, though, what do you say? What impact are technological developments having on our capacity for reproduction? In this piece, we examine how fertility varies with technological advancements and the ramifications for humans. We will talk about some of the ethical issues raised by the development of artificial intelligence (AI) and assisted reproductive technologies (ART), as well as their possible repercussions. Continue reading to find out more about the fascinating prospects that technology presents for reproductive health in the future.

It is noteworthy that developments in technology have brought about significant changes in fertility treatments in recent years. This is an overview of the state of fertility treatments today and how they are assisting individuals in becoming pregnant.

IVF Or In-Vitro Fertilization: IVF is one of the most popular and successful fertility treatments available today. It is a sophisticated sequence of operations intended to help with fertility or prevent genetic disorders and assist with childbirth. It entails taking the eggs out of the ovary, fertilizing them in a lab with sperm, and then putting the developing embryos into the uterus. IVF cycles typically last two months. Based on available statistics, approximately half of women under 35 will become pregnant and give birth after their initial IVF egg retrieval and subsequent embryo transfer(s). During the IVF process, preimplantation genetic diagnosis, screening, or testing for aneuploidy (PGD/PGS/PGT-A) can be used by intended parents to ascertain gender. These

chances will rise in tandem with increased AI infusion and learning, since several studies have indicated that AI has a promising function in decision-making to support diagnosis, prognosis, treatment, and much more.

Intracytoplasmic Sperm Injection (Icsi): ICSI is a kind of IVF that is performed when male infertility is severe.There are problems with the amount or quality of sperm. During ICSI, a single sperm is inserted into each egg. ICSI can be used even in situations where poor sperm quality has no bearing on infertility.After multiple attempts at in vitro fertilization have failed, some couples give ICSI a try. Documents show that, depending on skill, the success rate for ICSI can range from 85% to 90%. This indicates that with ICSI, 8 to 9 of every 10 eggs fertilized normally. ICSI cycles typically last four to six weeks to complete. For the egg and sperm retrieval procedures, the couple should plan to spend a half-day at the clinic. They should return two to five days later for the embryo transfer process. The goal of technological research is to thoroughly examine what functions and potential causes for the ease of repeatability.

Genetic Diagnostic Prior To Implantation (Pgd): One kind of genetic testing that can be performed on embryos before implantation into the uterus is called PGD. It can be applied to check for specific genetic flaws or illnesses. PGD has been used most frequently to treat single-gene illnesses, including Sickle cell disease, Tay-Sachs disease, Cystic fibrosis, and Spinal muscular atrophy (SMA). When one or both genetic parents carry a recognized genetic abnormality, it may be made available.

Assisted Hatching: IVF is occasionally used in this process. It entails creating a tiny hole in an embryo's outer layer so that it can readily hatch and integrate into the uterine lining. It is thought that assisted hatching may facilitate an embryo's implantation in the uterus, increasing certain patients' chances of becoming pregnant. Imagine what happens when all of the information gathered from different reproductive processes is examined to identify patterns and trends.

Cryopreservation Of Embryos: This method keeps embryos viable for use in the future. It frequently works in tandem with IVF to increase the likelihood of success. After being frozen, the embryos can be thawed and inserted into a woman's uterus. One method of preserving fertility is embryo cryopreservation. Frozen embryos can be safely preserved for ten years or longer, and are kept under observation at hospital facilities, typically a lab, or commercial reproductive medicine institutions.

In terms of reproductive treatments, technological advancements have been made recently. For couples who are having trouble getting pregnant, there are more options than ever, including in-vitro fertilization (IVF) and at-home ovulation kits.

Accessibility is one of the main ways that technology has improved reproductive treatments. Previously, a lot of couples needed to go to specialized clinics for treatment; but, these days, fertility clinics are opening up across the country. This implies that couples won't have to pay the additional expenses related to travel in order to get the care they require.

The cost of fertility treatments has almost completely decreased thanks to technology. Now, couples can increase their chances of success without incurring the costs of many IVF cycles.thanks to new developments including the ability to freeze eggs and embryos. This lessens the financial and psychological toll that fertility treatments can have on a person in addition to saving them money.

And lastly, technology has improved the efficacy of reproductive therapies. Because of developments in medical science, we now comprehend how conception functions and the variables that may affect it. As a result, new and enhanced treatment approaches have been created, aiding an increasing number of couples in realizing their goal of becoming parents.
Fertility treatments have a bright future ahead of them, but it's also full of uncertainties. While quick technological advancements are making it possible to develop new, more efficient reproductive therapies.

Nevertheless, the expense of IVF is high; a single round might easily exceed $10,000. IVF might also result in adverse outcomes like Ovarian hyperstimulation syndrome (OHSS) is a potentially harmful and uncomfortable condition.

A number of promising new treatments for infertility appear to be promising as technology develops. In vitro maturation (IVM) is one such procedure that includes taking immature eggs out of a woman's ovaries, developing them in a lab dish, and then fertilizing them with sperm.

IVM has been demonstrated to have a significantly decreased risk of OHSS while being just as successful as conventional IVF. A single cycle of IVM normally costs about $5,000, and it is far less expensive than standard IVF because it does not require strong medications to boost egg production.

Intrauterine insemination (IUI), which involves inserting sperm directly into the uterus, is another exciting new reproductive technique. It typically takes about two weeks following the surgery to ascertain whether the treatment is effective in the event that a pregnancy test is positive.

As technology develops, so does our comprehension of conception. We now understand that a number of factors might influence a couple's ability to conceive, and we are equipped with more resources than ever to support couples in overcoming infertility.

However, hope remains. Couples experiencing infertility can discuss their choices with their doctor and select the most appropriate fertility treatment. Many couples are able to conceive the child they've always desired thanks to modern treatment.

In conclusion, our understanding of fertility is growing along with technology. From comprehensive genetic analysis and at-home diagnostics to IVF procedures and newly technological technologies can provide us with unprecedented insights into our reproductive health.

Couples should keep up to date on the most recent developments in reproductive medicine and speak with their physician with any queries or worries they may have specific to their individual infertility process. Gaining more knowledge about your body's functioning will help you make wiser choices about conception, pregnancy, and raising a happy family.

It All Begins With The Egg:

Overview Of Assisted Reproductive Technologies (Art)

Art refers to medical interventions intended to induce pregnancy. Gametes, or eggs and sperm, are manipulated in these intricate therapies in order to enhance the likelihood of conception. People who may not respond well to other infertility therapies or those who have tried treatment but are unable to conceive may find that ART is a possibility.

Individuals who are thinking about ART frequently visit a medical expert about their alternatives and might need to see a fertility specialist.

While infertility is the main reason why individuals use ART, other people take it for genetic reasons or to prevent problems during pregnancy. ART may also be referred to as medically assisted reproduction or fertility treatment by some.

Due to the high cost of reproductive treatments like ART and their limited Medicaid and private insurance coverage, it could be challenging for many people to obtain them.

Varieties Of Art

Different techniques and reproductive cells are used in various types of ART operations. Which ART is best for a given situation can be determined by a doctor. In vitro fertilization is the most popular kind (IVF).

1) IVF

In IVF, eggs are extracted by a physician and fertilized in a specialized laboratory. Experts can combine this with in vitro fertilization-embryo transfer (IVF-ET), transferring the resultant embryos into the uterus of the patient. According to the Society for Assisted Reproductive Technology, 99 percent of ART operations involve IVF-ET.

The success rates of IVF treatments in 2018 for individuals utilizing their own eggs for a single oocyte retrieval are listed by the Centers for Disease Control and Prevention (CDC) as follows:

- 52% for those under 35 years old
- 38.1% of those in the 35–37 age group
- 23.5% of those in the 38–40 age group
- 7.6% of individuals over 40

An IVF success estimator (Trusted Source) is another tool that a person can use to calculate their chances of becoming pregnant after in vitro fertilization.

Some people may not conceive at all using IVF, and it may take more than one round to become pregnant. A higher likelihood of fertilization and pregnancy is one of the advantages of IVF. Possible side effects could consist of:

- multiple pregnancy, or the simultaneous implantation of two or more embryos

- adverse reactions to fertility medications, such as ovarian hyperstimulation syndrome

- ectopic pregnancy, in which the embryo implants extrauterine

According to the National Conference of State Legislatures, an IVF cycle typically costs between $12,000 and $17,000.

2) Intrafallopian Transmission
While some ART techniques are comparable to IVF, the gametes are delivered directly into the fallopian tube through laparoscopic surgery. Some may select this course of treatment because of their religious beliefs, or their insurance policy might only pay for this kind of ART.

Like other ART methods, there is a higher risk of multiple pregnancies. Furthermore, because the procedure involves a laparoscopy, there is a chance of surgical problems like infection, organ puncture, or anesthesia-related side effects. Generally speaking, intrafallopian transfers cost more than IVF.

Specialists rarely employ these procedures because of the higher risks and expenses associated with this type of ART. As a result, information regarding their success rates is scarce.

Types Consist Of:
- ➔ **Gamete Intrafallopian Transfer, Or Gift:** is a medical procedure in which a physician uses laparoscopic surgery to insert gametes directly into the fallopian tubes after gathering eggs and sperm in a tube. A person is not required to select which embryo to transfer because there is no IVF process.

- ➔ **Zygote Intrafallopian Transfer (Zift):** It is the combinationIVF and GIFT employing IVF techniques to stimulate and gather the eggs, specialists combine the eggs with sperm in a lab setting and then transfer the fertilized eggs, or zygotes, back into the fallopian tubes. ZIFT has the potential to help people become pregnant even if they have severe infertility problems or damaged fallopian tubes.

- ➔ **Pronuclear Stage Tubal Transfer (Prost):** It entails transferring a fertilized egg to the fallopian tube before cell division.

Transfer Of Frozen Embryos

In the United States, frozen embryo transfer, or FET, has grown in popularity. It entails putting previously frozen IVF embryos into a person's uterus after they have thawed. According to a 2017 study, 52% of FET recipients still had unfinished pregnancies.

The Human Fertilisation and Embryology Authority in the United Kingdom claims that FET is just as safe as using live embryos for medical purposes. On the other hand, some data points to a higher risk of preterm birth when using FET. Not every frozen embryo will survive the thawing out process, which is another potential risk associated with FET.

Although the price of FET varies, it can reach $6,000.

Intracytoplasmic Sperm Injection

Experts can use intracytoplasmic sperm injection (ICSI) in addition to in vitro fertilization (IVF) to aid in the fertilization of an egg. An embryologist, often known as an embryo specialist, injects a single sperm into the core of an egg using a tiny needle.

50–80% of eggs are fertilized by ICSI. ICSI has a success rate comparable to that of IVF, and for those whose infertility is caused by sperm, it might be a useful ART technique. ICSI will usually cost more than IVF because it is an add-on procedure to IVF.

Considerations Regarding ICSI Include The Following:

- Some or all of the eggs may be harmed during the process.

- The sperm injection may not cause the egg to develop into an embryo.

- There is a 1.5 to 3% probability that a kid born normally would have a serious birth abnormality. However, the birth defect might have been caused by the underlying infertility rather than the treatment.

Third-Party ART

A third-party ARTTrusted Source is a person or couple who receives an egg, sperm, or embryo donation from another person. Gestational carriers and surrogate mothers may also be included. These relate to situations in which an embryo from an ART-using couple is implanted in another person or inseminated with sperm from the couple.

Research indicates that 40% of transfers using donated frozen embryos from a 50%Trusted Source result in a live delivery and 50% result in pregnancy. Additional advantages of third-party ART consist of the following:

- When IVF has repeatedly failed, it might work.

- Avoiding passing on some conditions could be beneficial.

- It can benefit someone who has trouble carrying a pregnancy to term yet produces good eggs.

- It can benefit folks who struggle to produce sperm or eggs.

Third-party ART can be highly expensive, depending on the kind that individuals select. The least expensive method is usually sperm donation, which costs about $1,000 per vial.

Many cycles will require numerous vials, and the cost of a single vial for the other options can vary. The projected expenses are:

- $18,000–50,000 to donate eggs
- $13,000–17,000 for the adoption of embryos
- $60,000–150,000 for gestational carriers and surrogates

Getting Ready
One way to get ready for an ART treatment is to practice habits that could increase the likelihood that the therapy will be successful. This may entail making dietary adjustments, such as cutting back on alcohol and caffeine and taking supplements at the doctor's recommendation.

It can also entail giving up smoking and engaging in regular exercise. Prenatal careTrusted Source and tests can help maintain the health of the expectant mother and child when ART is effective.

Ethics
Several facets of ART give rise to moral questions, including:

- Does a single person or a pair require ART?

- Ownership of gametes and embryos that are stored?

- Is it moral for patients to contribute their eggs to a clinic in exchange for discounted or free care?

- How do various ART techniques fit with an individual's religious beliefs?

- Should ART be restricted based on age?

- Is it rightful for infants born by gamete donation to be aware of their origins and their biological parents?

- Are all ART requests handled the same way, regardless of a person's sexual orientation or relationship status?

- Is it moral to use frozen sperm or embryos from a deceased person?

How Innovations Like Ivf Can Aid In Conception

IVF, or in vitro fertilization, has advanced considerably in the last several years and is now a more practical choice for infertile couples. This development is attributable to continued innovation and research in the field of reproductive medicine. The most recent developments in IVF technology and how they are raising the prospects of success for prospective parents will be discussed.

An Overview Of The Most Recent Developments In Ivf Technology
1) Genetic Testing Prior To Implantation (Pgt): By choosing healthy embryos, PGT enables the screening of embryos to detect genetic problems prior to implantation, improving the likelihood of a successful pregnancy.

2) Temporal lapse Using Embryo Imaging: Continuous monitoring of embryo development utilizing time-lapse technology allows for better embryo selection based on growth patterns and milestones, enhancing IVF success rates.

3) Machine learning and artificial intelligence (AI): In order to optimize IVF results, AI and machine learning evaluate patient data and embryonic development to deliver individualized therapy suggestions.

4) Ovarian Tissue Cryopreservation: With the use of this technology, women receiving cancer treatment or other medical procedures that may impair fertility can freeze and preserve ovarian tissue that contains viable eggs.

5)Better Cultural Media: Improved culture medium formulations produce the perfect environment in the laboratory for the growth of embryos, increasing the quality of the embryos and improving the success rates of IVF.

6) Methods for Freezing Eggs: Women now have more alternatives for preserving their fertility because of the enhanced success rates of egg freezing achieved through vitrification, a quick freezing technique.

7)Transfer Of A Single Embryo (Set): By transferring a single, carefully chosen embryo, SET lowers the possibility of multiple pregnancies while maintaining high success rates and minimizing problems.

These developments signify the state-of-the-art methods and technologies that are revolutionizing the area of in vitro fertilization, raising success rates and elevating the patient experience in general.

Genetic Testing Prior To Implantation (PGT)

The growing use of preimplantation genetic testing (PGT) is one of the most noteworthy developments in IVF technology. Using PGT, embryologists can check embryos for genetic defects prior to implantation into the uterus. By identifying healthy embryos, this process lowers the danger of genetic abnormalities and increases the likelihood of a successful pregnancy. PGT is available in two primary forms: PGT-M (Monogenic) for single-gene diseases and PGT-A (Aneuploidy) for chromosomal screening.

Temporal lapse Using Embryo Imaging

With the use of innovative technology, time-lapse embryo imaging allows for ongoing observation of embryo development without requiring the removal of the embryos from the incubator's controlled environment. This enhances the selection procedure and success rates by enabling embryologists to identify the healthiest embryos based on their growth patterns and developmental milestones.

Machine learning and artificial intelligence (AI)

In the field of in vitro fertilization, artificial intelligence and machine learning have been introduced. To offer individualized treatment recommendations, these tools evaluate enormous volumes of data, including patient histories, embryonic development, and success rates. AI can assist medical professionals in making well-informed judgments, improving the likelihood of successful IVF treatments catered to the needs of specific patients.

Ovarian Tissue Cryopreservation

A breakthrough for women undergoing cancer therapies that could impair their fertility is ovarian tissue cryopreservation. With the use of this method, women can preserve and freeze their viable egg-containing ovarian tissue prior to receiving radiation or chemotherapy. There is hope for future pregnancies with the ability to re-implant the tissue after therapy is finished and the malignancy is in remission.

Better Cultural Media

There have been significant advancements in the culture media used to raise embryos in the lab. The optimal environment for embryo growth is provided by sophisticated culture medium formulations, which replicate the internal conditions of the female body. The result of this optimization is improved embryo quality and increased IVF success rates.

Methods for Freezing Eggs

Thanks to developments in freezing techniques, egg freezing, also known as oocyte cryopreservation, has become increasingly successful. Higher survival rates and improved egg quality when thawed are the outcomes of replacing the conventional slow freezing method with vitrification, a quick freezing process. For women who choose to put off having children for private or health-related reasons, this has increased their options.

Transfer Of A Single Embryo (Set)

In order to lower the possibility of multiple gestations and related problems, single embryo transfer (SET) is now the preferred method of IVF. With the advancements in culture media, genetic screening, and embryo selection, it is now feasible to transfer a single embryo with confidence, reducing the hazards involved in multiple pregnancies while preserving high success rates.

It All Begins With The Egg:

In Summary

The field of reproductive treatment is changing as a result of the most recent developments in IVF technology. Couples facing infertility have hope thanks to advancements in genetic screening, time-lapse embryo imaging, artificial intelligence, and improved culture medium. With every advancement in science and technology, there is a constant rise in the likelihood of IVF success, enabling more people and families all over the world to fulfill their ambition of becoming parents. It's critical to speak with a reproductive specialist if you're thinking about undergoing IVF therapy. They can walk you through your options and customize a treatment plan to fit your specific requirements.

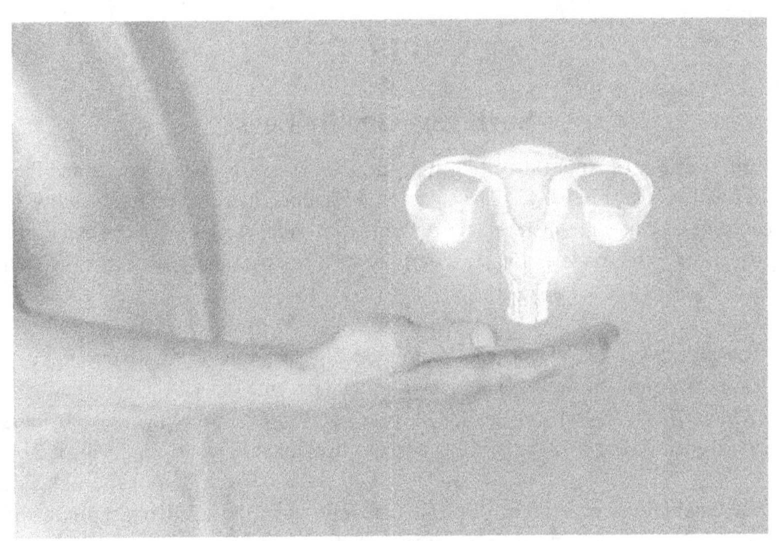

Chapter 3
Nurturing Quality Eggs

Chapter 3

Nurturing Quality Eggs

Fertility is a constantly fluctuating state, peaking at approximately age 35 and then declining noticeably at 45. The odds of difficulties increase and the ability to conceive can become increasingly difficult with time. According to research, the chance of miscarriage is rising as fertility declines. A significant factor in both cases is the individual's egg quality.

"The likelihood of miscarriage and infertility increases with decreasing egg quality.Women experience these things as they become older. Age, genetics, and environment all affect the quality of your eggs, says fertility specialist Aimee Eyvazzadeh, MD, MPH—a fertility specialist her patients call the "egg whisperer."

It's crucial to understand that although there are steps you may take to promote the health of your eggs, there is no foolproof method to alter the composition or quality of your eggs. "It's not fair to mislead women into thinking that egg quality is under our control," Dr. Eyvazzadeh observes. "We can control the things we eat and how we [lead] a healthy lifestyle...but that may not mean your egg quality will get better."

People can make decisions that may increase their fertility and support the quality of their eggs as they become more knowledgeable about their reproductive health.

Lifestyle Factors Influencing Egg Quality

We are all aware that a variety of aspects of our everyday lives are influenced by our lifestyle choices, but when was the last time you considered how your lifestyle may impact your ability to conceive?

Never—like many others, you may not see having children as your top priority right now—but do you plan to have kids in the future? Fertility is a long-term concern. When it comes to being ready to become pregnant in the future, it can be helpful to understand how your current lifestyle can affect your fertility. It could just be a minor adjustment or modification. You and your unborn child will both benefit from leading a healthy lifestyle.

Periodically - You most likely have plans to begin a family at some point in the far future.

Every day-It's likely that you are actively considering or preparing to start a family.

Numerous lifestyle factors, though not all-important, can affect your fertility now and in the future. These factors include stress, nutrition, BMI, alcohol and tobacco use, caffeine intake, and some medicines. Having said that, it's important to keep in mind that each person is distinct and varied, and this includes fertility.

Therefore, there is no one-size-fits-all method for treating fertility. Any person can make decisions that support a healthy lifestyle and tangentially increase both male and female fertility. Oocytes and spermatozoa, that is, need to be taken into account when analyzing how lifestyle factors may affect your chances of becoming pregnant. After all, it takes two to tango.

Numerous aspects of your daily life might be impacted by your lifestyle choice. Your overall mood and day-to-day energy levels are influenced by your nutrition and level of exercise. Your lifestyle decisions have an impact on more than just your mood and energy levels; they can also have an impact on your potential to become pregnant.

You can make the following lifestyle adjustments to enhance the quality of your eggs and your overall fertility.

1) Smoking

Fertility issues are more common in women who smoke. Smoking harms eggs, changes hormone levels, and prevents the ovaries from functioning properly, all of which have an adverse influence on the female reproductive system.

2) Alcohol

Consuming alcohol may also be detrimental to your ability to conceive. Alcohol may have a detrimental effect on hormone levels and, if you are already pregnant, may have an effect on the fetus's growth.

3) Caffeine

A small amount of caffeine has no effect on fertility, but if you consume 500 mg or more per day, it may negatively affect your ability to conceive. Ten espresso shots or five properly made cups of coffee are equal to 500 mg of caffeine per day.

4) Having Safe Sexual Relations Is Crucial.

It is thought that one of the main reasons for infertility is sexually transmitted infections. Chlamydia and gonorrhea are two diseases that can cause prostatitis, fallopian tube blockage, and other issues that lower fertility. It is always advised to use a condom during sexual activity because of this.

5) BMI

A higher or very low BMI might affect fertility in both men and women. Your BMI must be no higher than 35 to be eligible for private fertility treatment, and it must be no higher than 30 to be accepted as an NHS-funded patient.

Higher BMIs can affect sperm counts in men and women, hormone imbalances, pregnancy risks, and the quantity of medication required for fertility treatments.

6) Contraception

It isn't real! No kind of contraception—pill, IUS, IUD, injectable, ring, or implant—can cause infertility on its own. Medics, pharmacists, and nurses take proactive steps to prevent injury. They wouldn't recommend contraception that could render you infertile as a result.

7) Mental Well-Being

It's not an if-or-but situation. Fertility is a roller coaster of emotions. It is imperative that you take the time to accept that, despite your best efforts, you can't always avoid the tensions, anxiety, and stress that come with trying to become pregnant. Prioritizing your physical and mental well-being is something we strongly suggest doing when trying to conceive and during fertility treatment.

Patients frequently discover that talking about their ideas and feelings with others is facilitated by building a strong support system. Couples and individuals might benefit from including counseling into their reproductive journey by having a private space to discuss any emotions and discomfort they may be going through.

Nutrition And Its Impact On Fertility

i) Carbohydrates

Humans primarily utilize carbohydrates as fuel, which also control the glucose metabolic pathway and insulin-mediated glucose regulation. Carbohydrates can be simple sugars or monosaccharides, or they can be complex compounds such as certain oligosaccharides and polysaccharides found in plant cell walls. The values of the glycemic load (GL) and glycemic index (GI) indicate how carbohydrates impact blood sugar levels.

Consuming more complex indigestible carbs, including those in soluble dietary fiber or whole grain food products, will lower blood glucose levels. Increased whole-grain consumption has been linked to higher rates of live births and pregnancy. Likewise, eating more vegetables has been demonstrated to increase embryo quality following intracytoplasmic sperm injection (ICSI).

The consumption and metabolism of carbohydrates seem to control ovarian function as well. In fact, in the 2009 Nurses' Health Study II (NHS II), women who consumed more carbohydrates had an approximately 80% higher risk of ovulatory infertility compared to those who consumed the lowest quintile of carbohydrates.

It has been demonstrated that polycystic ovarian syndrome (PCOS) symptoms can be alleviated by following a diet that contains less than 45% of total energy intake from carbohydrates. This is achieved by elevating levels of follicle-stimulating hormone (FSH) and sex hormone binding globulin (SHBG), while lowering insulin and testosterone. In PCOS individuals who are overweight or obese, this is associated with decreased weight.

With a hypocaloric diet, in which half of the daily calories come from carbs, a greater number of ova were retrieved, and higher clinical pregnancy and live birth rates were reported in infertile and obese infertile women during IVF. But in addition to a decreased live birth rate, sugary soda consumption was also inversely associated with a lower number of ova recovered and embryos acquired by ovarian stimulation cycles.

ii) Proteins

Protein intake in a healthy adult is estimated to be 0.8 g/kg for every kilogram (kg) of body mass. Compared to plant proteins, consumption of animal proteins has been positively associated with ovulatory problems. It has been demonstrated that consuming 5% of energy from vegetable proteins instead of animal proteins can lower the incidence of ovulatory problems by over 50%.

Consuming dairy and soy has been linked to improved IVF results. This is due to the presence of phytoestrogens in soy, a class of isoflavones that resemble estrogen and have modest estrogenic action when they bind to estrogen receptors.

iii) Fats

Various food sources contain both omega-6 (ω-6) and omega-3 (ω-3) polyunsaturated fatty acids (PUFAs). Consequently, fish such as tuna, salmon, mackerel, and sardines as well as nuts, seeds, and plant oils are common sources of ω-3 PUFAs. On the other hand, chicken meat, fish, and eggs frequently include ω-6 PUFAs, which are also contained in nuts, seeds, and oils.

The effect of these fats on IVF outcomes has not been conclusively proven, but higher ω-3 PUFA consumption seems to be associated with improved pregnancy chances.

Nevertheless, certain foods like fish may raise the degree of exposure to persistent organic pollutants like methylmercury and dioxins. Similarly, vegetable and fruit intake may raise the risk of pesticide exposure.

Iv) Iron-Rich Vegetarian Foods

Like whole grains, legumes, spinach, fortified cereals, and long-grain enriched rice. To improve the absorption of iron, include vitamin C in your meals in the form of berries, bell peppers, and citrus fruits.

Patterns of the "Fertility Diet"

A 2007 study titled "Fertility Diet" by a group of Harvard researchers indicated that women with ovulatory infertility who adhered to this dietary pattern had a 27% lower risk of infertility from other sources and a 66% lower chance of ovulatory infertility.

- More monounsaturated fat (found in foods like avocados and olive oil) and less trans fat

- Increased vegetable protein and decreased animal protein

- More foods high in fiber, low in glucose, and high in carbohydrates (including whole grains)

- Less meat and more vegetarian sources of iron

- Multiple vitamins

- Higher fat dairy as opposed to lower fat dairy

Generally speaking, you can meet your nutrient needs and maintain a healthy weight by eating a variety of vegetables in sufficient proportions, opting for monounsaturated fats rather than saturated and trans fats, eating at least half of your grains whole, and consuming enough calcium-rich foods, including dairy.

Remember to Take Folic Acid

It is important that women who are trying to conceive have enough folic acid, even if it won't make them more fertile. In order to prevent neural tube malformations, folic acid is required. Three to four weeks after conception, before most women even realize they are pregnant, the neural tube grows into the brain and spine. The U.S. Preventive Services Task Force (USPSTF) has recommended a daily supplement that contains 400 to 800 micrograms of folic acid in addition to eating foods high in folate and folic acid, like fortified cereals and dark leafy green vegetables. See your doctor first if you're thinking about taking dietary supplements.

Healthy Habits For Optimal Reproductive Health

Adopting a few healthful habits can sometimes be the key to getting pregnant. Perhaps all you need to do to improve your chances of getting pregnant is make a few dietary and lifestyle adjustments. When combined with a specialist's advice, you can create a healthy daily routine and increase your chances of becoming pregnant. These practices will continue to improve your health even after you get pregnant.

Here are a few healthy practices you can adopt to maintain optimal reproductive health.

1. Schedule Regular Examinations For Gynecology

Everybody should get a yearly gynecological checkup in order to diagnose and treat diseases affecting the female reproductive system as soon as possible. During the examinations, conditions including cervical cancer, menstruation issues, pelvic pain, sexual dysfunction, and urine leaks were identified.

To identify your illness, the doctor may do a pelvic exam, Pap smear, or ultrasound during the check-up. Getting the greatest prenatal care might also be a smart start if you intend to become pregnant.

2. Keep Your Diet Balanced

Choosing healthier foods on a daily basis is the most important thing you can do to enhance your reproductive and general health. To learn more about the foods that will work best for you and increase your chances of getting pregnant, speak with a dietitian.

You can incorporate whole grains, fruits, vegetables, and foods high in omega-3 fatty acids into your everyday diet. You also need to abstain from processed foods and sugar-filled beverages.

3. Avoid STIS, Or Sexually Transmitted Infections

Many STI types have a significant impact on women's reproductive systems, increasing their risk of vaginal infections, pelvic inflammatory disease, genital ulcers, and infertility. You must avoid these dangerous illnesses if you want to keep your reproductive system healthy.

By always engaging in protected intercourse, you can avoid STIs. When having sex, you should always use condoms appropriately and practice good hygiene to stop the spread of illnesses. In order to avoid STIs, you may also go to the top gynecologist hospital in Siliguri and get the necessary immunizations.

4. Maintain A Healthful Body Mass

Obesity and excessive body weight are linked to infertility and poor reproductive health. This is due to the fact that obese women are known to overproduce the hormone leptin, which can result in a hormonal imbalance.

The entire functioning of your reproductive organs, including your menstrual cycle, will be disrupted by improper hormonal systems. Among the actions that can be performed to maintain a healthy body weight are eating a balanced diet, getting regular exercise, and adhering to appropriate sleeping schedules.

5. Control Your Stress

Stress can cause problems with menstruation, including missing periods or delayed ovulation, by interfering with the ovaries' and the brain's normal connection. To enhance reproductive functioning, you must be able to control your stress through the use of relaxation techniques, communication, and handling sexual stress.

When you call a gynecologist in Siliguri, he might also recommend some additional supplements, such omega-3 fatty acids and folic acid, to help with ovulation. It's also possible to maintain a healthy reproductive system by cutting back on coffee, restricting intense activity, and quitting smoking.

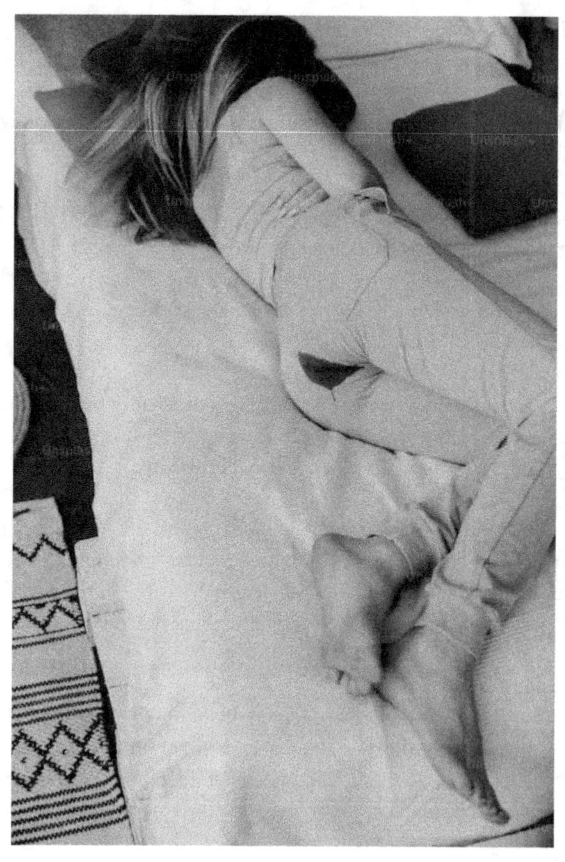

Chapter 4
Overcoming Odds and Avoiding Miscarriage

Chapter 4

Overcoming Odds and Avoiding Miscarriage

A miscarriage, which is technically referred to as a spontaneous abortion, is the death and ejection of a pregnancy before it is able to survive on its own. Miscarriages are the term sometimes used to describe all kinds of pregnancy loss including pregnancies that terminate in abortion before 20 weeks of gestation.

ESHRE defines miscarriage prior to 6 weeks of gestation as a biochemical loss. Clinical miscarriage is the term used when ultrasound or histology evidence indicates the presence of a pregnancy; it might be "early" before 12 weeks or "late" between 12 and 21 weeks. A stillbirth is another term for fetal mortality that occurs beyond 20 weeks of gestation.

Understanding Common Causes Of Miscarriage

First trimester
In the first trimester, miscarriages account for about 80% of cases. The interval between weeks 1 and 13 is referred to as the first trimester.

Frequent Reasons For Miscarriages In The First Trimester Are:
- **Anomalies In Genetics**: Chromosome issues in the fetus account for more than half of all first trimester miscarriages. Your body will terminate the pregnancy if it determines that the fetus is damaged or has missing chromosomes.

- **Blood Clots:** caused by antiphospholipid syndrome (APS) have the potential to terminate a pregnancy. Medication is a treatment option for this illness in order to avoid miscarriage.

- **Ectopic Conception:** This rare but possibly dangerous kind of pregnancy develops when the fetus starts growing outside the womb. Ectopic pregnancies are medical emergencies that need to be treated right away since they cannot be saved.

- **Placenta Problems:** The pregnancy could end if the placenta and fetus are incompatible. Similarly, abrupt pregnancy termination can also result from uterine abnormalities, such as an irregular shape.

Second Trimester

During weeks 13 to 24, the later stages of pregnancy, miscarriages are substantially less prevalent. If it does happen, the mother's health issues or other external health concerns are most likely the cause.

Frequent Reasons For Miscarriages In The Second Trimester Are:

- **Infection:** An infection in the cervix or uterus can cause miscarriage. Similarly, food-borne infections can increase a woman's chance of miscarrying.

- **Persistent Ailments:** A woman's chance of miscarriage is increased by long-term health issues such as diabetes or high blood pressure. If the problem is not adequately controlled or treated, the risk increases.

- **Illness Of The Thyroid:** The chance of miscarriage increases with untreated thyroid problems.

- **Autoimmune Conditions:** Miscarriages can result from autoimmune diseases like lupus and others.

- **Issues Pertaining To The Cervix Or Uterus:** Unusual womb shape or fibroids might result in miscarriage.

- **Lifestyle Factors:** Alcohol consumption, drug usage, smoking, and secondhand smoke can all affect a fetus's development. Excessive intake of caffeine could potentially be harmful.

- **Environmental Factors:** Miscarriages can occur as a result of exposure to specific chemicals or risks. These consist of heavy metals, paint thinners, solvents, insecticides, and mercury. There is also evidence connecting air pollution to a higher risk of miscarriage.

It All Begins With The Egg:

Third Trimester

A miscarriage at this late stage of pregnancy is most often referred to as a stillbirth. Pregnancy loss in the third trimester can also be caused by the same problems that lead to miscarriages in the first two trimesters. However, pinpointing the precise cause is frequently challenging.

These problems could consist of:

- **Complications Throughout Pregnancy:** This covers premature labor as well as placenta dissociation.

- **Birth Defects:** 10% of stillbirths are the outcome of a congenital abnormality that is either structural or genetic.

- **High Blood Pressure:** Of all pregnancies, 5 to 8 percent end in preeclampsia. Preeclampsia can rob the fetus of oxygen and nutrition, but the mother bears the majority of the risks associated with this illness. Additionally, preeclampsia can develop into eclampsia, a dangerous illness that can kill both the mother and the fetus.

- **Uncontrollable Diabetes.**

- **Infection:** The pregnancy may terminate due to an infection in the fetus or placenta.

- **Issues Related To The Umbilical Cord**: This chord can stop the fetus's blood and oxygen supply if it is knotted or compressed.

- **Issues With The Placental System:** An inadequate blood supply to the placenta may result in miscarriage.

Strategies To Reduce The Risk Of Miscarriage

1) Establish Good Habits Before Getting Pregnant

You're already halfway to building a sound foundation if you can start preparing for pregnancy before conception, even though it's not always possible. According to Stephanie Zobel, MD, an OB-GYN at Winnie Palmer Hospital, "up to half of

Because pregnancies are not always planned, some parents may not be at their best when they do get pregnant.

planning a family. United States Department of Health and Human Services, n.d.

While many women do not become aware that they are pregnant until a few weeks after they miss their period, Dr. Zobel continues, by then the fetal spinal cord has already developed and heart activity can be felt.

This is a gentle reminder that if you're planning a pregnancy, there are things you can do to promote a healthy pregnancy even if you're one of the many individuals who didn't discover you were pregnant for several weeks.

"Dr. Zobe states that it is best for all pregnancies to prepare for pregnancy by changing diet and exercise, reducing stress, improving chronic medical conditions, and starting prenatal supplements. To help reduce the chance of some congenital defects that may also be linked to miscarriage, use a prenatal vitamin that contains at least 400 mcg of folic acid.

2) Arrange For A Preconception Examination
Make an appointment for a preconception checkup with an OB-GYN or other healthcare practitioner if you are not currently pregnant. In addition to reviewing your medical history and getting a sense of your lifestyle, they will do an annual examination (if one is needed). Additionally, blood samples will be taken to test for Rh factor, blood type, and immunity to diseases like rubella and varicella.

Pregnancy is the ideal time to receive vaccinations against infectious diseases if you have not already developed natural protection from an infection. These vaccines are live viruses that cannot be administered once you become pregnant, but missing them won't make you more likely to miscarry. However, if you are exposed to the viruses while pregnant, they can protect you and your unborn child.

3) Consume a Nutrient-Dense, Balanced Diet
Even though you may already be taking a prenatal vitamin, it's not a panacea. According to Dr. Nichelson, the best method to receive the vitamins and nutrients

your body needs to sustain your body and your pregnancy is to eat a balanced, nutrient-dense diet. There is some indication that there may be a connection between specific nutritional deficits and pregnancy loss, even if studies on the exact relationship between nutrition and miscarriage are conflicting.

Furthermore, you should stay away from items that increase your chance of contracting foodborne illnesses like listeriosis, or an infection caused by the bacteria Listeria, which can result in miscarriage, an early birth, or stillbirth.Six Raw meat and shellfish, raw milk and dairy products, undercooked eggs, raw sprouts, and deli meats are among the foods on this list.

4) Moderate Exercise

When you find out you're pregnant, you should keep up your regular fitness regimen, even though it's not the time to begin training for your first marathon or begin a new, strenuous exercise regimen. Moderation and adhering to exercises your body is accustomed to are crucial.

Although the precise relationship between extremely high and intense physical activity and early pregnancy loss is unclear, some research points to this possibility. Contact sports are also prohibited for the time being since they may cause an injury or fall that could harm the developing fetus. Make sure you obtain permission from your healthcare physician before beginning any new fitness program while you are pregnant.

5) Limit Caffeine Intake

The American College of Obstetricians and Gynecologists' official position is that while there is no conclusive evidence linking caffeine consumption to miscarriage, pregnant women may wish to limit their daily intake to no more than 200 milligrams, or about two 8-ounce cups of regular brewed coffee. Ask your prenatal care provider what they recommend if you have any concerns about caffeine use, as there is some evidence linking high levels of consumption to bleeding in the first trimester.

6) Steer Clear Of Alcohol, Tobacco, And Recreational Drugs.
Dr. Zobel advises women who may become pregnant to cut back on or avoid
drinking altogether. She adds that people who use recreational drugs or smoke
should speak with their doctors about getting help quitting, as these behaviors may
be associated with a higher risk of miscarriage. Although there are currently no
reliable human studies demonstrating that marijuana use during pregnancy might
result in miscarriage, there may be a connection, particularly in the first trimester,
based on research on animals.

7) Seek Assistance in Handling Stress
Effective stress management may benefit not only your general mood but also the
general health of your pregnancy. According to a 2017 Scientific Reports analysis
of the literature, stress may raise the risk of miscarriage by as much as 42%.

However, bear in mind that regular stress or worry isn't associated with the loss of
a pregnancy, according to Jonathan Schaffir, MD, an assistant professor of
obstetrics and gynecology at Ohio State University College of Medicine. Major
stressors such as divorce, abuse, or experiencing another kind of loss or grief are
the source of the issue. Discussing options for therapy or medication with your
doctor can be beneficial if you are facing a lot of stress in your life.

8) Control Chronic Illnesses Like Diabetes
Pregnant women with diabetes should seek help and take care to manage their
disease as best they can, as high blood sugar can result in fetal deformity and a
subsequent loss, says Dr. Nichelson.Thirteen

If at all feasible, it is important to visit a doctor in order to maximize your health
before getting pregnant. "Chronic medical disorders including diabetes,
hypothyroidism, hypertension, and autoimmune illnesses need to be addressed and
well-controlled prior to pregnancy," in line with Dr. Zobel. "For women with
long-term medical issues, seeing a doctor early in the pregnancy is essential to a
favorable outcome.."

9) Consult Your Physician About Low-Dose Aspirin.
After one or two miscarriages, are you attempting to become pregnant again?

It All Begins With The Egg:

According to a 2021 study that was published in the Annals of Internal Medicine, taking "baby" aspirin at a low dose may assist avoid having another miscarriage.14 More pregnancies, live births, and fewer miscarriages were linked to study participants who took one 81-milligram tablet daily during their infertility and pregnancy—as long as they followed the aspirin regimen religiously.

Naturally, not everyone attempting to conceive will benefit from using a blood thinner, so before incorporating medicine into your daily regimen, make sure to consult a healthcare professional for additional advice.

10) Examine Your Current Medication

Make sure the medication you take, even over-the-counter remedies, is safe for pregnancy by consulting an OB-GYN or other healthcare provider before using it. For instance, ACE inhibitors, which are cardiac drugs, can result in fetal abnormalities and raise the risk of miscarriage.15 That being stated, avoid abruptly quitting any medications you take on a regular basis since this may also result in health issues. Always discuss drug changes with your doctor before beginning or ceasing.

Pregnancy and infertility are the safest times to avoid certain medications, but others should be carefully considered after weighing the advantages and risks. Consult your doctor before making any changes to your medication before or during pregnancy, since there are situations when it may be best for some women to continue taking mental health medication in order to have a safe pregnancy.

11) Hands Washing.

Numerous infections can result in stillbirth, miscarriage, or the death of the unborn child. The best defense against contracting any of these bacterial or viral infections is to wash your hands frequently and keep your distance from sick people and congested indoor areas.

Good Hand Hygiene

- Use warm water and soap to wash your hands for at least 20 seconds, or as long as it takes to sing your ABCs twice. Wash everything always:

- both prior to and following meals

- Following a bathroom visit

- After handling objects that other people have handled, such as cash, doorknobs, pencils, or shopping carts, or after being near someone who is ill.

12) Give Up Smoking

Smoking poses a serious threat to health. It raises your risk of heart disease, high blood pressure, stroke, lung illness, and several types of cancer. Individuals who smoke, or are exposed to secondhand smoke, have an increased risk of miscarrying, stillbirth, preterm delivery, low birth weight babies, and infertility.5.

Sudden Infant Death Syndrome (SIDS) is more common among babies born to smokers. Giving up smoking could ensure that you live long and happy years as a parent in addition to saving the life of your unborn child.Six

13) Exercise Caution In The Kitchen:

Food-borne infections such as listeria are linked to a higher risk of miscarriage. It is standard practice to advise pregnant women to stay away from foods like undercooked meats and unpasteurized cheeses that are known to be the most frequent sources of harmful bacteria. To prevent diseases, however, appropriate food handling is even more crucial than usual.

Food Safety

- Make sure you cook eggs, fish, and meat to the proper temperature.

- Store leftovers in the refrigerator as soon as possible.

- Wash fresh produce very well.

- Meat and fish should be consumed or frozen one to three days after purchasing.

- Both before and after handling raw food, wash your hands.

14) Obtain A Flu Vaccine

Despite the widespread belief that receiving the flu shot increases the risk of miscarriage, numerous studies have shown no such correlation. It is advised to receive an inactivated influenza vaccine regardless of the stage of pregnancy.

Pregnant individuals are particularly vulnerable to the H1N1 strain, which has a higher fatality rate than the general population.8 Neural tube abnormalities in the fetus are also linked to a high temperature during pregnancy.

Pregnant women who have COVID-19 may become sicker than normal and have a higher chance of preterm birth.10 Avoid catching the virus by taking preventative measures, such as donning masks indoors and being vaccinated to lower your risk of developing a serious infection.

15) Strive For A Balanced Weight

Similar to smoking, obesity has been connected to a host of health issues. These include a higher risk of heart disease, diabetes, and some cancers, as well as pregnancy complications include gestational diabetes, preeclampsia, early birth, and miscarriages of any kind. Additionally, being underweight raises the possibility of miscarriage and other pregnancy-related issues.

The entire explanation for the association between fat and miscarriage remains unclear to experts. However, research from all around the world is producing similar findings. Obese women are more likely to experience miscarriages.
Despite the widespread belief that receiving the flu shot increases the risk of miscarriage, numerous studies have shown no such correlation. It is advised to receive an inactivated influenza vaccine regardless of the stage of pregnancy.7.

Pregnant individuals are particularly vulnerable to the H1N1 strain, which has a higher fatality rate than the general population.8 Neural tube abnormalities in the fetus are also linked to a high temperature during pregnancy.9.

Pregnant women who have COVID-19 may become sicker than normal and have a higher chance of preterm birth.10 Avoid catching the virus by taking preventative measures, such as donning masks indoors and being vaccinated to lower your risk of developing a serious infection.

16) Have Safe Sex

While it may seem absurd to advise safe sex to individuals who are trying to conceive or are already pregnant, STDs such as syphilis and chlamydia can actually increase the risk of miscarriage, stillbirth, neonatal mortality, infertility, ectopic pregnancy, low birth weight, and other complications.

A sexually active person is susceptible to STIs. When you begin prenatal care, you will be screened; however, if you or your partner have more than one sexual partner, you might wish to get examined even before you start trying to conceive. Even if you are pregnant, you should use a condom if you have more than one partner. You should also wait to use condoms with a new partner until you have both undergone STI screening.

17) Abstain From Alcohol

Due to the possibility of fetal alcohol syndrome, pregnant women in the United States are recommended not to drink alcohol. However, regular or heavy alcohol consumption increases the chance of miscarriage or stillbirth.17

There is no proven lowest safe level of alcohol consumption, thus it is best to refrain completely during pregnancy. Other countries have different recommendations regarding the amount of alcohol use that is safe. See a healthcare professional about this if you drink frequently or don't think you can stop, and try to limit your intake of alcohol.

Coping With The Emotional Challenges Of Pregnancy Loss

It is typical to experience a range of intense feelings, including shock, numbness, grief, sadness, guilt, rage, and a sense of vulnerability and failure, after losing a baby, regardless of the infant's developmental stage.

As soon as the pregnancy test result was affirmative, you started your path towards motherhood. Maybe you had fantasies about the baby's appearance and, naturally, about what it would be like to be their mother. Though the loss dashes these hopes, grieving and loss processing is a personal path, much as how each woman experiences pregnancy is different.

These six suggestions should aid you in your grieving journey.

1. Recognize That It's Not Your Fault
Following a miscarriageBecause many OB/GYNs do not educate women about the likelihood of miscarriage, pregnancy loss or complications are more common than you may assume.

In the aftermath of a pregnancy loss, individuals frequently attempt to make sense of what went wrong by trying to figure out why it happened. They frequently wonder what they could have done—or not done—differently or differentially to have avoided the situation, but in all likelihood, there was nothing you could have done to change the outcome.

One in every four women experience an early miscarriage, with the majority occurring in the first trimester as a result of a chromosomal abnormality, or an error in the baby's chromosomes. One miscarriage occurs in five pregnancies by the second trimester, which lasts between thirteen and nineteen weeks.

Although prevalent, these losses are frequently imperceptible. Women frequently lose their babies to miscarriages early in pregnancy, usually before they have even told anybody they are pregnant, therefore they frequently don't receive much assistance during their grieving process. Well-meaning individuals frequently underestimate the intensity of grief a loss can evoke, even when they are aware of the pregnancy.

A stillbirth occurs when a pregnancy ends beyond 20 weeks; the likelihood of this occurring is reduced to about 1 in 160 pregnancies. We know that there is no predictor of who will be impacted by stillbirth and who won't, but for about half of stillbirths, the cause can be analyzed. This indicates that in over 50% of cases, the cause cannot be found.

The conclusion to be drawn is that, despite having done "everything right" and having meticulously planned your pregnancy, you are not at fault and were unable to stop your loss from occurring.

2. Recognize The Grieving Process You Are Experiencing
We don't actually move through the phases of grief in a linear fashion; rather, each stage builds upon the one before it. The initial stage of the mourning process is typically denial, or "This isn't happening, this can't be happening," during which you may feel numb until your mind is able to begin understanding what has happened. Usually, people swing back and forth between the phases for as long as the mind needs to.

Anger could then follow, maybe aimed at your loved ones, the medical staff, or even at your own body. I frequently hear women in my private practice who work with miscarried women express anger against their bodies for "letting them down" and for being unable to perform tasks that other women seem to perform with ease. or enraged at partners who don't get how much of a sense of loss they are experiencing, or at medical personnel they felt weren't helpful.

During the **bargaining stage**, our minds begin to work out why the miscarriage occurred and what we could have done to avoid it. I could have prevented this if I had done xyz. This stage is closely associated with guilt and anger, but keep in mind that pregnancy problems and loss are not your fault; nothing you did or did not do caused this to occur!

When someone starts to admit to themselves that they have lost something, they may desire to isolate themselves from everyone (depression stage) and experience feelings of hopelessness, grief, sobbing, guilt,and inadequacy.

And lastly, **acceptance.** You are no longer preoccupied with the events of the past, despite your anguish at remembering them. But please keep in mind that acceptance doesn't happen in a certain amount of time. Allow yourself time to recover. Do not force yourself to move on from your sadness too soon. Give yourself permission to process your grief when it arises.

We have a shared past with that individual, complete with pictures and recollections of the times you two had together, and we grieve for them when they pass away. The loss of the narrative in which you imagined the characteristics of your future kid and yourself as a mother is one way that grieving a miscarriage differs from other types of grieving. I believe that the medical community and society at large frequently fail to acknowledge the breadth of emotions that a miscarriage can cause. This may intensify a woman's sense of loneliness and her conviction that she should move on swiftly.

3. Make An Effort To Keep A Social Circle Open.

Don't face the world straight after your loss if you don't feel ready to. Taking a little break from work to take care of yourself is perfectly acceptable. But after a while, try not to isolate yourself from other people.

Despite the fact that talking about it could hurt, telling others about your experience will make you feel less alone and promote healing. You may be astonished to learn how many of your friends, neighbors, coworkers, and even family members have also suffered personal losses if you feel comfortable sharing what has happened.

It's unlikely that someone who has never experienced loss can truly understand what it's like to miscarry. The majority of people want to provide consolation, yet they may be at a loss for words or even come up with something patronizing like "You're young; you can always try again." When someone says something incorrectly or, in certain situations, says nothing at all because they are at a loss for words, try not to take it personally.

Tell folks straight out about what you need. You might need to avoid talking about it if you are out with friends or back at work because you are afraid you won't be able to control yourself. Thank them for their sympathies, but tell them you can't talk about it right now. Instead of holding all of your sentiments within, talk to someone about your feelings—either in a support group or with a friend who can relate.

In order to process and come to terms with your grief, as well as to help you deal with the challenging feelings you're going through right now, you might also want to look for a therapist who specializes in pregnancy loss.

4. Take Care of Your Physical Needs

It's crucial to take care of your physical health because your body is fragile at this time, even if it feels like everything is confusing and melancholy makes it impossible to do daily things like eating and sleeping. In addition to healing from the numerous hormonal and physical changes brought on by pregnancy, you are also grieving. After a stillbirth, your body will experience the same hormonal and physical changes as if you had given birth, therefore your physical recuperation and healing may take longer.

The amount of pregnancy you had before the loss does not, in my opinion, affect the feelings of sadness and loss you experience afterwards. Eating a balanced diet, staying hydrated, and getting enough sleep are all essential for maintaining your physical health, which allows you to concentrate on your mental well-being.

5. Putting Your Emotions In Writing Can Help

The brain attempts to make sense of a terrible incident that someone has experienced, but if thinking about your loss is upsetting, you may be trying to ignore the thoughts. However, try not to push your emotions away because doing so will simply cause them to fester and occasionally surface as anxiety or rage. Make time in your schedule to reflect on and analyze the experiences you have had or are having. Keeping a journal is one method for doing this.

Writing in a diary is a terrific method to explore your emotions and sentiments, and since it's private, you can be honest with yourself about your thoughts and feelings without feeling the need to edit them.

Research has indicated that journaling during depressive episodes helps expedite the healing process. If you are having trouble putting the past behind you, it may

It All Begins With The Egg:

help to schedule a brief time each day—once or twice—to examine your feelings in your notebook before closing it. When ideas cross your mind outside of journal writing time, tell yourself that you don't want to worry about them right now and that you will address them later in the day. This creates mental boundaries to prevent you from dwelling on what has happened and its possible implications all the time.

Pick a spot where you won't be disturbed for fifteen minutes, or for whatever long you choose, to write in your journal. If you find it difficult to start or believe you might not enjoy writing, give yourself five minutes, and use that time to write in notes or bullet points. Grammar, spelling, and sentence structure are unimportant.

Try to be conscious of your thoughts and feelings around your loss when you write, and keep in mind that you are in control of this process and that there is no right or wrong way to go about it—you just need to pace yourself. Ease up and write about something else if you are feeling very upset until you are ready to delve deeper once more.

Remain aware of the present moment and try not to let your thoughts wander to potential future events, especially those that could be disastrous.

After a writing session, expect to have unpleasant feelings. However, if you have been sitting for a long time without moving, try taking a short stroll or cleaning the kitchen while listening to your favorite song.

6. Recognize That Ptsd And Anxiety Can Develop Following A Loss
We have talked about the emotions that can surface during the grieving stages and are aware that the majority of women experience some level of psychological distress following a miscarriage or stillbirth; however, for certain individuals, the symptoms of anxiety and/or depression are more persistent and can seriously impair their ability to function.

After A Pregnancy Loss, Common Signs Of Anxiety And Despair Can Include:
- Angry or furious outbursts or a depressed mood for the majority of the day

It All Begins With The Egg:

- Absence from friends, family, and other social interactions

- inability to get asleep and remain asleep

- Embarrassment, guilt, and inadequate feelings

- inability to focus and make judgments

- Using unhealthy coping mechanisms to deal with stress, including binge drinking or overeating

- pondering over what has transpired

- Investing too much time in the internet to learn about miscarriage and other health issues

Generalized Anxiety Disorder (GAD): After a pregnancy loss, it is sometimes associated with worries that a future pregnancy may again result in loss and suspicions that there may be an underlying medical or genetic problem that contributed to the loss.

Acute Stress Disorder (ASD): is a condition that develops within hours of a stressful occurrence (the loss of pregnancy), and it lasts for at least two days but no more than four weeks. Acute stress disorder symptoms can include:

- a feeling of detachment or insensitivity to emotions

- Feeling disoriented or detached from oneself

- Unable to remember specific details of the trauma

- Reliving the incident via persistent dreams, flashbacks, or thoughts

- Keeping things out of the way that bring up the miscarriage

- Continuous nervousness and/or anxiety

While the duration of PTSD symptoms is longer than four weeks, they are similar to ASD symptoms.

- invasive reliving of a painful prior event (perhaps the birthing itself in this instance)

- Nightmares or flashbacks that may concern the moments just before, during, or after childbirth

- avoidance of stimuli related to the occurrence, such as sensations, ideas, people, locations, and specifics of the incident (usually involves avoiding medical facilities, hospitals, periodicals about childbirth, and other new mothers)

- Chronically high levels of arousal (agitation, restlessness, hypervigilance, heightened startle response)

- Panic episodes and anxiety

- experiencing a sense of disassociation and unreality

The degree of ongoing psychological suffering can equally affect women who have had an early miscarriage or stillbirth, and it is unrelated to the number of weeks a person was pregnant. An intriguing study from the Imperial College in London discovered that after three months of follow-up, 28% of the 186 women who had lost an early pregnancy satisfied the criteria for PTSD.

It's critical to keep in mind that you are not alone in experiencing ongoing anxiety, depression, or stress disorders, and that getting expert care can truly help you move forward. Recovering from a loss is not about forgetting what happened; rather, it's about acknowledging that it happened and resuming your life's activities, free from the grip of the past or future.

I hope this information has been useful to you as you begin your healing journey. Taking care of your mental well-being is just as vital as your bodily well-being. When you're ready, allow yourself to grieve, accept your feelings without blaming or criticizing yourself, and seek assistance by speaking with other women who have also lost a pregnancy.

It All Begins With The Egg:

Although each person's journey is unique, please give yourself time to come to terms with what has happened and lament what could have been. Do not be afraid to seek professional assistance if your worries, depression, or trauma reactions are interfering with your day-to-day activities and you feel trapped. In the event that you do not reside in one of the states where I have a license (Florida or Illinois), your physician can connect you with mental health providers in the area who specialize in treating trauma and grief brought on by miscarriage and stillbirth.

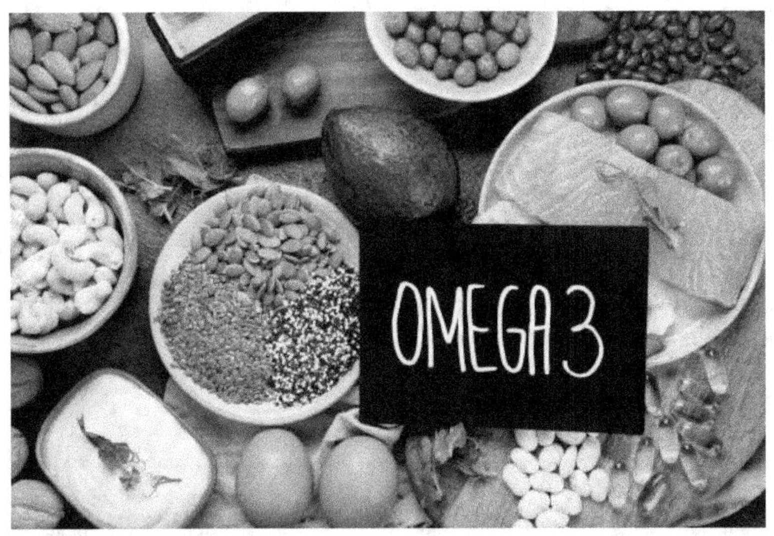

Chapter 5
Natural Approaches to Improve Fertility

Chapter 5

Natural Approaches to Improve Fertility

Natural approaches to improve fertility refers to approaches that can be used in getting pregnant naturally—that is, without the use of fertility treatments or other supports.

There are natural strategies to boost a woman's and a man's fertility. Unfortunately, a lot of men and women lack the knowledge and awareness necessary to improve their chances of becoming naturally pregnant.

Holistic Methods For Enhancing Fertility

It is quite feasible to conceive naturally. All you need is knowledge and advice on how to increase fertility by occasionally making small adjustments to your way of life and approach, as well as how to become pregnant naturally.

Natural Pregnancy Method

1) Let's Start With Your Physical Well-Being
Being physically fit is the first step toward becoming pregnant and having a safe pregnancy. Being overweight or underweight can have a detrimental impact on fertility and the ability to have healthy children.

Make sure you work out three or four times a week. Because it increases lung capacity and blood circulation, aerobic exercise is vital. Yoga poses help improve balance and posture, while weight-bearing workouts help you build muscle and reduce weight more quickly. All of this helps you become healthier, which raises your chances of getting pregnant and having a safe pregnancy.

Your treatment of your body is the foundation of your physical wellness. Exercise is a great way to stay in shape during pregnancy, but it's even more crucial to make sure you're not doing anything that could harm your chances of getting pregnant

It All Begins With The Egg:

and having a healthy baby. It's critical that you give up any bad behaviors or habits that compromise your bodily well-being.

To optimize your well-being, you ought to get rid of or minimize the following:

- Smoking
- Recreation Drugs
- Alcohol
- Dangerous Substances
- Coffee

Make sure you discuss any prescription drug you take with your healthcare professional. It can be dangerous to use some drugs while pregnant. To improve your chances of conceiving and having a healthy pregnancy, your doctor might decide to stop treating you or change the medications you are currently taking.

Furthermore, maintaining regular intake of specific nutrients and vitamins, as well as eating nutritious, well-balanced meals, is directly tied to your overall health and wellness. For more beneficial suggestions, read our piece on preconception nutrition and health for men and women.

2) The Ovulation Process
Understanding when ovulation is happening is one of the secrets to simple conception. Ovulation predictor kits or fertility monitors can be used to track ovulation. But, without the use of these kinds of kits, you can naturally track and forecast when you will ovulate.

The calendar approach should allow you to monitor your ovulation if your cycle is regular and lasts 28 to 32 days. All you have to do is mark the first day of your most recent menstrual cycle on a calendar and determine the day of your subsequent menstrual cycle. Once you have that, you will be able to count back eight or eighteen days and determine the day ovulation will occur. Ovulation happens on a single day between cycle days 11 and 21 in an average 28-day cycle (29-day cycle, 12–22 days; 30-day cycle, 13–23 days; and so on).

A secondary method of tracking ovulation involves observing alterations in your cervical mucus. Your mucus will become more pliable, slick, and stretchy as ovulation approaches. It is frequently likened to egg whites. This alteration is directly linked to ovulation, and you should ovulate on the day you detect the greatest amount of this discharge of egg whites.

To monitor your basal body temperature, you can also use a basal thermometer. Immediately following ovulation, your basal body temperature will increase.
These methods of naturally tracking your ovulation are a part of a family planning approach known as natural family planning, or fertility awareness (NFP). The article Fertility Awareness has further information regarding basal body temperatures, cervical mucus, and the calendar technique.

3) Timing Intercourse
Some attempt to schedule their sexual activity for just before or during ovulation. Although this can be effective, there is a better way for those who are trying to conceive to manage their sex schedule. You should be able to use a standard fertile window to schedule sex if your cycle is regular and occurs every 28 to 32 days.

You should be aware that, for the regular cycles mentioned above, ovulation usually takes place between day 11 and day 21 of the cycle. The majority of individuals are unaware that sperm can remain inside of you for two to five days after sexual activity. To find out when you are fertile, check our free ovulation calendar.

When the sperm, or semen, is already inside and waiting for the egg to be released, the odds of conception are at their highest. Here are some tips on how to approach your sex routine and step up your efforts to conceive based on the facts provided.

Ten days should pass after the start of your most recent menstrual cycle. For the following ten days, have sex today and every other day. You can increase your chances of receiving healthy, mature sperm during each sex session by scheduling sex every other day. On this plan, sperm will be added during ovulation and semen will be placed within until the egg is expelled.

It All Begins With The Egg:
67

4) Nutrition

Your physical health is intimately correlated with your diet. But healthy pregnancies and fertilization are also related to nutrition. Eating meals that are well-balanced and rich in the necessary vitamins and nutrients is crucial for overall wellness and good health. This is one of the most crucial actions for a healthy you that is directly tied to the health of your fertility when combined with exercise.

The proper daily consumption of fiber, protein, carbs, and vital fats should be your focus. In addition to consuming a balanced diet, there are certain essential nutrients that support the health of your reproductive system and facilitate natural conception.

The importance of folic acid during the first few weeks of pregnancy cannot be overstated, even though it is more closely linked to the development of a healthy fetus than to fertilization. To avoid neural tube abnormalities, make sure you are getting 400 to 800 mcg of folic acid each day.

5) Vitamins, Nutrients, And Nutritional Aspects

The following is a summary of some of the essential vitamins, minerals, and nutritional components you should always have in your diet:

i) Water: Consuming water promotes hormone balance, maintains organ function, and aids in the removal of pollutants from the body. All of this works together to boost your fertility.

ii) Complex Carbohydrates: Consuming fruits, vegetables, and whole grains gives you the fiber and nutrients that boost fertility while also assisting your body in eliminating toxins through water-soluble absorbents.

iii) Protein: Consuming protein helps you become more fertile by supplying nutrients that aid in the creation of hormones. Red meat, however, need to be restricted and lean. Diets heavy in red meat may cause endometriosis issues.

iv) Fatty Acids: Consuming nuts, seeds, and oily fish, such as salmon and mackerel, is an excellent method to receive fatty acids, which help both the development of your unborn child and your own fertility.

It All Begins With The Egg:

v) Whole Milk: Consuming whole milk has an impact on your ability to conceive. According to research by Chavarro and Rosner, women who drank three glasses or more of whole milk each day had a 70% lower chance of experiencing ovulation failure and becoming infertile.

vi) Zinc: Deficits in zinc have an adverse influence on both men's and women's fertility. Enhancing fertility in both men and women can be achieved by taking 15 mg of zinc daily. Vegetables, eggs, whole grains, peas, onions, beans, and more contain zinc.

vii) Vitamin B6: Consuming this vitamin on a daily basis supports the regulation of progesterone and estrogen and aids in the generation of the female sex hormone. Eggs, salmon, peanuts, bananas, and soybeans are foods high in vitamin B6.

viii) Vitamin C: Vitamin C promotes a healthy sperm count and motility in men and helps women ovulate. Vitamin C is found in a variety of fruits and vegetables, including oranges, blueberries, and strawberries.

ix) Vitamin E: Taking vitamin E has advantages for both men and women. For women, this vitamin influences hormone function; for men, it improves sperm quality.

6) Keep Them Relaxed And At Ease.
Men who wear tight underwear are less likely than those who wear loose underwear to produce immobile sperm.Because they must be kept at a lower temperature for the best sperm generation, testicles hang from the body.

It is believed that this is due to the testicles' little but noticeable rise in warmth brought on by their extended proximity to the body.

Approximately one in four infertile couples receive a diagnosis of "unexplained infertility," meaning that there are no known medical causes for the failure to conceive. We must investigate whether psychological and emotional elements are the root of the issue if physiology is not the issue.

In the clinic, it is frequently observed that, even in cases where there are established physical variables, recognizing and treating underlying unresolved difficulties can be the crucial element in paving the path for a successful pregnancy.

Obstacles might stem from a variety of concerns, such as anxieties about changing bodies, giving birth, or how having a kid will affect your employment. They could also result from traumatic prior events like sexual abuse or miscarriage.

A professional with training in hypnosis and psychotherapy for improved fertility can assist you in exploring and resolving unresolved issues so they are no longer stored in your body and do not prevent conception. This can also change the emotional and psychological effects that attempting to get pregnant or having fertility treatment has on you.

Thus, the greatest strategy to increase your fertility is to keep your testicles colder by taking cold baths and showers, avoiding direct heat, wearing loose-fitting clothes like boxer shorts, and choosing clothes that leave plenty of space around your genitalia.

Mind-Body Connection In Fertility

Your body goes through physical reactions to every idea you have and every emotion you experience. The Mind-Body connection is the idea that your thoughts have an impact on your physical health.

According to a Harvard study, women who participated in mind-body fertility programs had a 52% chance of becoming pregnant, compared to a 20% chance in the control group. These women also experienced more than TWICE the likelihood of becoming pregnant, increasing their chances of becoming pregnant from 1 in 5 to 1 in 2.

In today's episode, we'll break down the specifics of how a mind-body fertility program might increase your chances of getting pregnant, in seven different ways.

It All Begins With The Egg:

The extra benefit of a Mind Body Program, however, is something I want to discuss with you first. It's not only a tool to help you conceive; it's also a tool to help you FEEL BETTER, control your stress levels, and reclaim your happiness (something I can't say is true for fertility clinics). However, when paired with assistance from your fertility specialist, it can be the hidden weapon and game-changer for maximizing the success rates of IUI and IVF.

What Is A Mind Body Program?
The relationships between the brain, body, mind, and behavior are the main emphasis of mind-body practices. They are there to support you in managing your reaction to stressors in your life, especially emotional ones, and helping you comprehend how your body is interconnected so that you may control how your body is responding physiologically. This can entail bringing bodies back into a parasympathetic or relaxed state through mental or physical movements and acts.

Then, in what specific ways does a Mind Body Program enhance fertility?

1. It Improves The Equilibrium Of Your Hormones.
Most of our hormones are produced or released by the hypothalamus (and frequently by the pituitary gland) in response to the activation of either the sympathetic or parasympathetic nervous systems. Imagine this as your brain's command center, distributing impulses throughout your body. The problem is that when our sympathetic nervous system is active, our bodies prioritize producing cortisol at the expense of other hormones. It also doesn't prioritize or transmit hormones to our reproductive organs. When our bodies are given the option, they will always select cortisol over another substance. Therefore, we can more effectively balance our hormone production once we can enhance that process.

2. They Assist You In Making Wiser Choices
Our Prefrontal Cortex, which is in charge of making decisions, solving problems, rational thought, and impulse control, shuts down when our bodies are overly engaged in our fight-or-flight sympathetic nervous system, which becomes lodged in our limbic system, the emotional center of our brain. We are better equipped to evaluate the situation and decide what is in our best interests when we can get back there.

It All Begins With The Egg:

3. They Lessen Behaviors That Undermine Oneself.

When you are in a state of extreme stress, it can negatively affect your motivation, self-talk, self-confidence, and ability to adapt. This can lead to self-sabotage, which can be caused by eating a diet that is too restricted, over supplementing, or lacking in nutrients. It is much easier to not only make logical decisions but also to carry out our plans when we are able to modify the way our brains interpret and respond to specific circumstances as well as how we experience the events as they actually are.

4. Enhances Sleep

Hormone disruption caused by sleep deprivation can also have an impact on other aspects of our lives. Research has indicated that sleep has an impact on our immune system, reproductive hormones, appetite hormones (a sleep deprivation has been linked to desires for processed and high-energy meals), and nighttime crying intensity. You can learn techniques and methods to help you fall asleep more easily and stay asleep through the night with the support of a mind-body fertility program. (I frequently encounter women who wake up at 3 a.m. and are unable to get back asleep; this is generally due to an imbalance between cortisol and melatonin.)

5. We Can Reorganize Our Dominant Neural Pathways With Its Assistance.

Our brain uses neural pathways to transmit messages, but it can also have dominant neutral pathways. These pathways, which we can visualize as a well-traveled path through a forest, tell our amygdala to overreact and set off our fight-or-flight response, making it seem as though it takes less and less for us to become highly emotional and triggered.

6. Improved Advocating For Oneself

A Mind Body Program focuses on mental exercises and methods that can increase our ability to think clearly and boost our self-esteem. These two benefits when combined can increase our confidence in our ability to follow our gut instincts and make the changes that are best for us, which will increase our chances of getting pregnant.

7. Technical Instruments For Stress Management
One of the main advantages of a Mind Body Program is that it can teach you how to be less reactive to stress and give you tools to help restore homeostasis (balance) in the event that you do trigger your fight or flight response. Stress is an inevitable part of life and will continue to affect us through various challenges in our lives. One of the primary issues facing modern society is not only that stress exists, but also that there is no definitive conclusion to it, in contrast to prehistoric times when, for instance, if we managed to escape a tiger, our bodies would clearly sense the threat and start to heal. A Mind-Body Program can teach us how to physically calm our bodies and manage stress.

Alternative Therapies And Their Role In Conception

Holistic approaches to natural and integrative methods of addressing fertility problems and advancing reproductive health are provided by alternative therapies. We'll look at a range of complementary and alternative treatments that may improve general health and raise the likelihood of conception.

1) Herbal Treatments to Boost Fertility
For ages, herbal medicines have been utilized to promote reproductive health and manage issues related to conception. Actually, a number of "natural fertility boosters" have stood the test of time. Many herbs haven't yet been the subject of reliable clinical trials, nevertheless. Because of this, you should speak with a licensed herbalist and your doctor before using herbs in your regimen. Herbs can have a variety of effects, so it's vital to take any potential drug interactions into account.

2) The Acupuncture's Power
The traditional Chinese medicine of acupuncture has grown in acceptance as a substitute treatment for infertility. This method of controlling energy flow, or "qi," entails inserting tiny needles into predetermined bodily locations. The theory behind acupuncture is that by bringing the body's energy pathways back into balance, it can improve reproductive health. Research indicates that acupuncture may lessen stress, increase the likelihood of a successful conception, and improve

blood flow to the reproductive organs. Numerous couples find solace in the calming and harmonizing effects of acupuncture, while research is still in progress.

Beyond its physiological effects, acupuncture has potential benefits for enhancing conception. Acupuncture offers a holistic approach that includes emotional well-being in addition to its physical benefits. Hormonal balance and general reproductive function can benefit from the relaxation and stress reduction that acupuncture sessions provide. Acupuncture generates a peaceful, emotionally balanced environment that serves as a favorable environment for conception. It's important to note that acupuncture has become more popular as a complementary therapy to traditional reproductive treatments, even if individual results may differ. Acupuncture can be a useful tool for couples navigating the frequently difficult path to parenting because of its possible physiological effects and ability to boost emotional resilience during the reproductive process.

3) Meditation And Yoga For Fertility
Because stress throws off the hormonal balance and interferes with ovulation, it can have a major effect on fertility. Couples are realizing this and using mind-body techniques like yoga and meditation to improve their chances of getting pregnant. Yoga is a centuries-old technique that offers poses that improve pelvic blood circulation and encourage strength and flexibility. On the other hand, meditation provides an effective means of calming the mind, lowering anxiety, and enhancing emotional health. Couples can support their mental and physical health and foster a conducive environment for conception by adopting these techniques into their daily routine.

4) Diet's Function In Enhancement
Our reproductive health is just one aspect of our overall health that is greatly influenced by what we consume. Fertility can be supported and hormonal balance optimized with a nutrient-rich, well-balanced diet. Nutritional decisions can affect the general environment for conception, the regularity of menstruation, and the health of eggs and sperm. Foods high in antioxidants, whole grains, and leafy greens are frequently advised because they may improve the quality of eggs and sperm. On the other hand, cutting back on processed meals, coffee, and alcohol can

increase fertility. It is advised to speak with a dietitian for individualized advice based on fertility objectives.

5) Chiropractic Treatment and Embryology
Traditionally linked to musculoskeletal health, chiropractic care has drawn interest as a different strategy for enhancing fertility. The focus of this therapy is on nerve system function and spinal alignment, which may have an impact on reproductive health. Spinal misalignments may interfere with nerve signals that regulate the reproductive organs, therefore compromising fertility. The goal of chiropractic adjustments is to return the nerve system to normal, which may enhance reproductive health. Some people have claimed success when combining chiropractic care with traditional fertility therapies, but additional research is required.

6) Drug Use's Effect on Reproductive Health
Whether prescribed or recreational, drug use can have a serious negative effect on your reproductive health and interfere with your plans to become a parent. Both illegal substances and some prescription pharmaceuticals have an impact on fertility. They may upset ovulation and sperm production, tamper with hormonal balance, and adversely impact general reproductive health. Alcohol, smoke, and recreational drugs are examples of substances that can lower fertility by changing hormone levels and lowering the quality of eggs and sperm.

Certain prescription drugs meant to treat chronic illnesses may unintentionally influence fertility by altering the function of reproductive organs or generating hormonal imbalances. It's critical to understand that your decisions about drug usage may have long-term effects on your potential to become pregnant and have a healthy pregnancy. It's best to speak with a healthcare provider if you're hoping to increase your fertility so you can learn about the possible risks of drug use and look into other choices that will support your reproductive health.

7) Accepting Holistic Routes to Parenting
Making the decision to become a parent by using complementary and alternative therapies to increase fertility can be gratifying and powerful. Individuals and couples can maximize their reproductive health and raise their chances of naturally

It All Begins With The Egg:

conceiving by taking care of their body, mind, and spirit. But, especially for people with underlying medical concerns, it's critical to pursue these therapies with reasonable expectations and in combination with medical counsel.

A comprehensive strategy for enhancing fertility may involve incorporating herbal treatments, acupuncture, yoga, meditation, nutrition, and chiropractic adjustments into one's daily regimen. These treatments improve mental health and fortify the mind-body link in addition to its physical advantages. Keep in mind that every person's journey is different, and what suits one person might not suit another. To develop a thorough strategy customized to each patient's needs, open discussion with holistic practitioners and healthcare specialists is essential.

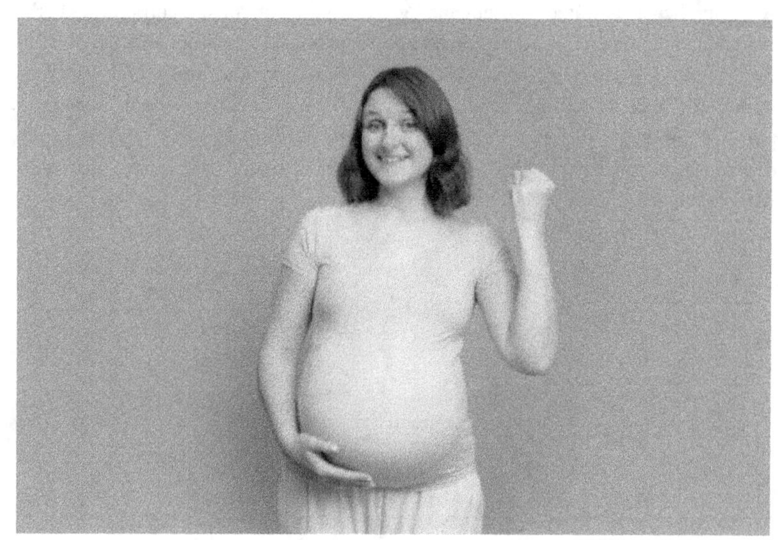

Chapter 6
Pregnancy Triumphs

Chapter 6

Pregnancy Triumphs

Zain Rajani, who is 22 days old, was born using a novel technique based on the finding that women may be able to overcome infertility brought on by low-quality eggs within their own ovaries. pristine stem cells from undeveloped, healthy eggs that can help a woman's older eggs behave more youthfully. These precursor cells can only grow into eggs, in contrast to other types of stem cells that can become any type of cell in the body, even malignant ones.

At First Steps Fertility in Toronto, Canada, where she resides, Zain's mother, Natasha Rajani, 34, underwent a brief laparoscopic operation in May 2014 to remove a little portion of her ovarian tissue. After identifying and removing the egg stem cells, scientists from OvaScience—the fertility startup that provides Augment—purified the cells in order to harvest their mitochondria.

The energy centers of cells are called mitochondria, which act as a molecular battery to power every cell function. The IVF outcomes were significantly enhanced when the mitochondria from these egg precursor cells were added to Natasha's low-quality eggs and her husband Omar's sperm. Natasha laid fifteen eggs in the Rajanis' first standard IVF effort, but only four of those were fertilized and only one of those progressed to the point where Natasha's physician felt safe transferring it. "I understood it wasn't the greatest embryo, but it was hers," she adds. First Steps Fertility's Dr. Marjorie Dixon.
Two of the four embryos that Rajanis created have been frozen in case the couple decides to have further children. Zain, the infant, was born to another.

Real-Life Examples Of Overcoming Fertility Challenges

Fertility is a marathon, not a sprint, so we must arm ourselves with all the strategies available to us so that we can successfully navigate this obstacle in our lives. Being diagnosed with infertility does not preclude you from becoming a parent. It is true that many people have encountered infertility at some point in their lives; it is defined as trying for a year without success. Some people

It All Begins With The Egg:

overcome infertility and go on to have children naturally, while others will require therapy.

We want to provide or draw attention to some advice on how to overcome every obstacle that infertility may present . Stress levels associated with infertility are high, and the condition affects many facets of a person's life, including self-perception, relationships with partners, and outlook on life in general. However, there is hope and a treatment that works for everyone.

Even if your circumstances can feel overwhelming at times, you need to understand how to lessen the tension that goes along with it. One thing we must acknowledge right away is that infertility is an emotional rollercoaster; therefore, feelings are affected not because you are weak but rather because you feel overburdened. The first thing you should know is that this is quite normal. It is critical that you recognize your emotions and realize that everything you are going through is completely normal. Particularly in a setting like ours where having children is highly valued.

Being parents has long been a dream for many couples, and now infertility is threatening that dream. We hardly ever seek professional counseling in this setting since it may be so emotionally and physically taxing. Although everyone thinks they are strong, infertility will put your strength to the test. Thus, consulting a therapist is not a sign of weakness. You need someone to talk to if you haven't been doing that. That somebody may be your partner, but you may occasionally need to see a professional counselor. It should be acceptable for you to express your worries and inquiries.

Strategies To Overcome Infertility Challenges

- It's crucial to surround yourself with knowledgeable individuals, which is why having a clinic is so crucial. The people you converse with in your clinic hold great significance. Fertility treatment is not a case of wishful thinking. You need someone who can both understand and respond to your questions and concerns. That's where getting expert assistance is also helpful. Fertility groups can also be helpful because they contain individuals who are experiencing similar issues to your own. They are able to communicate with you and comprehend your perspective. It is crucial that you make use of these kinds of groups. It is crucial that you join peer groups, but use caution as well. As with most things, you should be aware of the credentials and experience of the individuals who are in charge of these groups.

- Allow yourself to be furious and cry from time to time. Don't try to suppress your grief, guilt, or rage. Do not hesitate to cry if that is how you feel. Please stay in your room and punch your pillow if you feel like it. Feel free to cry if you need to about how unfair it is to get pregnant again or have a difficult pregnancy. Avoid attempting to suppress your emotions. You shouldn't feel guilty for how infertility affects your emotions; these reactions are perfectly natural. You should be aware that you should always seek expert assistance if you feel that you are unable to handle the situation any longer.

- Please remember to acknowledge the process, and let go of your sadness while you give yourself permission to breathe. As you can see, the counseling we are used to in this setting is church counseling, where the pastor is the expert on everything. This isn't the case for fertility or professional counseling, which is why some individuals get dissatisfied because it's not the counseling they're used to. For example, in church counseling, your pastor is able to respond to questions you pose. However, a competent counselor lets you come up with a solution on your own. Because you have to know what your own circumstances are. It's possible that couple A and couple B will go through distinct experiences. Therefore, if you were to provide everyone with the identical solution, it would be problematic. In most cases, the counselor only asks questions to help you comprehend the ramifications of your treatment decisions; you come up with the answer when you work through counseling.

- Additionally, it is preferable if you have a journal or notepad on which you can record your emotions. Write down your experiences. Maintaining a journal has the benefit of being readily available at all times. Writing down your thoughts is always an excellent method to let off steam. If necessary, write down your feelings and address them later. One thing infertility does is make you feel alone, so if you feel like you need to talk to someone about it later, you can always do that. That's why it's always a good idea to keep in touch with loved ones during this time. Maintaining a relationship with your loved ones is crucial. You can inform them about your preferences for treatment, even if they have never experienced infertility. Tell them how you want to be treated, and explain to them why some comments are insensitive even when they are made accidentally.

- You have to get better at communicating with your spouse. Without a question, infertility can strain your relationship and cause conflict between you two. If you master coping mechanisms, infertility can strengthen you too. Infertility has strengthened several couples. Never forget that there's a chance you two won't always agree on everything. Unless you deliberately align yourselves, as the two of you would react differently in a crisis. Thus, it follows that communication is crucial. Even if that means getting counseling together to ensure that you are in agreement. Since your partner is the person you are closest to, it is crucial that you both understand each other. Don't put yourselves apart because this individual knows exactly what you're going through because they are experiencing the same thing as you. Refrain from letting infertility break you.

- You and your partner must spend time together as well. Have fun together; it doesn't have to cost a lot of money. Proceed to the cinema if you are forced to do so. Your life shouldn't be ruined by infertility. You should do whatever it is that keeps you going, whether it's playing or taking walks—just make time to spend time together. It's crucial to safeguard your sexual life as well. Don't only have sex to procreate—enjoy each other while you can.

- You also need to educate yourself. Since infertility entails a great deal of uncertainty about the future, knowledge truly is power. Investigate on your own, then describe your condition and potential courses of action. For instance, you need to be able to determine your success rate for your age. I frequently say that treating infertility is not wishful thinking. You can't just walk up to me at 48 and tell me you want to use your eggs because someone told you that was acceptable. Compile your homework, learn as much as you can about the circumstances, and consult with subject matter specialists. By doing this, you shield yourself from inaccurate information and greatly facilitate the process of making wise decisions.

- You need to figure out what works best for you when it comes to reducing stress. Some have mentioned that walking, praying, meditating, and even visiting a therapist are helpful. Thus, you have the option to practice yoga, join a support group, or even learn more about your circumstances. Simply engage in whatever de-stresses you. Just be sure you are doing everything correctly, and breathing exercises are one more thing you may do. It can be done anywhere and is reasonably priced. Both by yourself and with your partner are viable options. All you have to do is take a comfortable seat and close your eyes. Draw in a deep, leisurely breath. Breathing in through your nose and out through your mouth is possible. You inhale deeply into your chest and then slowly release the air. This can be continued for around five minutes, and it can help you feel calmer.

- Your nutrition is another crucial factor to consider. What you consume matters since you need to maintain your body's health when dealing with issues related to infertility. You must follow a healthy diet in order for your BMI to be normal. Reduce your intake of white flour, sugar, salt, and saturated fat. You may also wish to cut back on the usage of technical food additives, such as alcohol, in your meals.

11 Things to Quit If You Are Facing Fertility Challenges
Suffering with infertility is not easy. Having said that, we can occasionally exacerbate our own problems. Naturally, not knowingly or purposefully. We can be unaware that there are other options. Or perhaps we're not even aware that we're undermining our own efforts.

1) Give Up Blaming Yourself
Perhaps you waited "too long" to have children. Perhaps you experienced problems conceiving because of something stupid you did while you were a college student.

It All Begins With The Egg:

Perhaps you're wondering whether it wasn't the best decision to survive only on fast food that year.

Alternatively, it's possible that you are clueless about what caused your current infertility issues. You know, though, that if you had known better, you could have stopped it.

Stop putting the blame on yourself. You should quit blaming yourself even if you can find a way to make it "your fault." It is ineffective. You get depressed from it.

Furthermore, the majority of infertility instances are unpredictable or not avoidable. It's really impossible to predict whether you would become a Fertile Myrtle or not if you had done something else. Let go of the guilt and concentrate on what matters most at this moment: making progress and solving the issue.

2) Give Up Hoping For A Sign
If you are over 35 and have been trying to get pregnant for more than a year (or more than six months), and you are not successful. It's time to consult a doctor if you have been trying to conceive for more than a year (or more than six months if you are over 35) and you are not successful. However, some couples decide they aren't the right fit for this advice. It's for those other people. The infertile ones, you know. They choose to hope for a miracle and carry on trying on their own.

The issue with that line of reasoning is that certain reasons of infertility deteriorate over time. Your chances of receiving your miracle might be dwindling the more you pray.

There's nothing wrong with opting not to seek fertility treatment in the end or even with choosing to keep trying while waiting for treatment. However, you shouldn't shun fertility tests. If nothing else, at least learn what's wrong and what your options might be.

Make sure that whatever is ailing you and your spouse can wait by getting checked out. Next, you might choose to have a "miracle waiting" period. Ask your doctor how long they believe you can try before you lose too much time.

It All Begins With The Egg:

83

3) Quit Feeling Optimistic

An infertility diagnosis can be devastating. It can be challenging to look beyond the upcoming few days or weeks at times. It's possible to feel despondent and convinced that you'll never become pregnant or have a happy existence.

If you are unable to conceive naturally, you may be able to use an egg, sperm, or embryo donor. Consider adoption if donor gametes are not an option. If adoption is not an option for you, keep in mind that happy, normal lives can be had without children.

To be clear, the pain does not magically disappear because of these alternative options. It will take time for you to process your loss and recover from the trauma of infertility.

But when you begin to doubt your ability to become pregnant or when you begin to believe that your life is over, do everything in your power to cling to a glimmer of hope. After infertility, there is life. Please keep that in mind.

Even if it's possible that you won't get pregnant, if you can keep your mind on the bright side of things, you'll feel better. For many couples, low-tech therapy are effective. You might be more likely to succeed than you believe. Consult your physician regarding the specific prognosis for you.

4) Quit Being Helpless

The majority of couples take very proactive care of one another. Nevertheless, not everybody is aware that they make the decisions.

To the couples who have been trying for more than a year yet are told by their doctors that they are "too young,"

Refusing to consider the possibility that the clinic may not want to "ruin" their reputation by using a risk, are the couples whose fertility clinics declined to attempt in vitro fertilization (IVF) using their own eggs due to low possibilities...

To the ladies whose doctors won't test or treat them unless they reduce weight, but leave it to them to figure out how exactly to do it...

It doesn't seem like you're that powerless. Go see another doctor if the one you are currently seeing won't perform an evaluation. If a clinic declines your application on the grounds that your odds are "too low," get a second opinion.

If your physician advises you to reduce weight, make sure they assess and address any hormone abnormalities that can make weight loss challenging. You should also get a recommendation to a nutritionist. Perhaps go seek a second opinion to see whether losing weight is truly necessary before anything else.

You are far more powerful than you think. Never be reluctant to defend your own interests.

5) Give Up Living in Two-Week Bits
This is a simple one, yet it happens so often that it is worth mentioning. Your life can easily divide into two-week periods when you're trying to conceive: the two weeks you spend waiting for ovulation and the subsequent two weeks spent waiting to get a pregnancy test.

The worst thing about this is that there are no breaks—that is, no period when you can relax and not worry about when you're going to ovulate or about getting pregnant.

Even if it's impractical to expect yourself to just stop worrying, you ought to make an effort to get past the crazy two-week wait period. To learn how, you might require the assistance of friends, a support group, or a counselor. However, it is feasible.

6) Give Up Determining Your Worth by Fertility
You may feel unworthy when you are infertile. shattered. Feeling embarrassed. Men and women who deal with infertility frequently feel all of these things.

It All Begins With The Egg:

Prior to beginning your infertility journey and realizing you were infertile, you most likely had a different, ideally more optimistic, self-perception. Keep in mind that the previous version of yourself still exists. When you are told you are infertile, you do not change into someone else.

If you were already amazing and lovable prior to becoming infertile, you continue to be such after becoming infertile. If you have any doubts, consider what you would say to a friend who confided in you that they felt useless and humiliated by their infertility. It's unlikely that you would tell them, "Yes, you're correct. You have no value at all!" Not in a manner.

You need to realize that it's not true of yourself, just as you know it's not true of a buddy. Your fertility is just one aspect of who you are.

7) Quit Viewing Sexuality as Broken
From passionate to tedious, sex can change. When trying to conceive, sex might become a reminder of your infertility.

You probably considered sex to be more than just a way to get pregnant before you tried to conceive. But after you battle with conception, for some reason, sex becomes a malfunctioning conception machine.

It's possible that everything you formerly enjoyed, including the connection, desire, and warm sentiments, would go.

Remind yourself that having a child is not the sole aspect of your sexual life. Prior to beginning your reproductive quest, list all the pleasures you derived from having sex. Try to bring some of it back into the bedroom if at all possible. You can enhance your sexual life while attempting to become pregnant, however it will require some effort.

8 Give Up on Wishing to Be a Family.
The notion of what constitutes a true family in society is rather narrow. Ads lead us to believe that in order to be considered real, one must have two children and a dog.

Family is, in fact, defined in a variety of ways. To be eligible, you do not need to be related by blood, have kids, or own a dog.

A couple facing infertility may decide to start their own family customs or holiday traditions after they become parents. They worry that they won't be able to continue those pleasant customs till they have their own children because of how their houses were while they were growing up.

That is untrue. You can come to regret the time you wasted if you put off starting a family. Begin your family's life now. If you don't wait until you have two children and a dog, the real family police won't come knocking on your door.

9) Give Up Trying to Be Your Own Person
Your life extends beyond your kin and your significant other, of course. You lead a separate life as well. Difficulties with fertility can cause you to lose perspective.

It's simple to stop thinking about your school or profession when you're experiencing infertility. Infertility-related stress can make it challenging to focus at work, which is detrimental to one's ability to pursue professional goals.

Having said that, it's worthwhile to stand back and evaluate your professional objectives. Are there any goals you formerly had but have since abandoned or forgotten?

There is more to your life than just your job. Your hobbies are listed there. Your overall health-related behaviors. Your connections.

Whether you're trying to conceive or not, and whether you eventually become pregnant or not, the years will pass. Recall to make the most of your time on Earth. Give getting pregnant less of your attention and allocate some of it elsewhere. Remember to enjoy the remaining years of your life.

10) Give Up Suffering in Silence
Though it's a possibility to think about, you generally shouldn't disclose your infertility difficulties to everyone. However, keeping it all under wraps is not only

It All Begins With The Egg:

needless but also emotionally taxing.

Something like that festers when you keep it a secret. The guilt you feel about your illness keeps getting worse. Shame grows best in dark places, just like mold.

Telling even one friend about your infertility difficulties will help to alleviate some of your shame.Think carefully about the friends and relatives you believe can be of help, and share your thoughts with them.

Don't let it stop you if the person you inform has a negative reaction. Until you discover someone with whom you can truly be yourself, try someone else. Not having to keep it all inside will be a relief.

11) Give Up Trying to Finish This by Yourself
You are not alone in this vast world, despite the fact that you could feel alone and that you seem to be the only infertile couple among all your friends. At some point in their lives, one in eight people will struggle with infertility.

Like you, there's a strong chance that someone you know has experienced difficulties conceiving, but they are choosing to remain silent about it. Break the silence with courage. You are unaware of how many options you have for assistance.

A RESOLVE infertility support group is open for you to join. It is possible to join the fertility forum. You can join the vast fertility blogosphere by starting an infertile blog. You can locate a therapist who can guide you through the challenging feelings associated with infertility.

Make sure you ask your partner for support as well. It's incredible how two individuals may experience infertility together as a pair and still attempt to manage it independently.

Talk to one another. Talk to each other about all of your fears, including the serious ones, such as concerns that you won't be able to conceive and your spouse will leave you. Depend on one another. See a therapist jointly to address any issues that have arisen as a result of infertility in your relationship.

The Joy Of Achieving A Natural Pregnancy After Fertility Struggles

Trying to conceive (TTC) is the only thing that can make you feel more alone and stressed. Anxiety is common when you're ready to start a family and things are difficult, even if you may have spent a lot of time up until now trying everything to avoid getting pregnant.

These conception stories may inspire you when you're feeling down, even though there isn't a simple solution for how to become pregnant.

It Took Two Years To Become Pregnant.
Ashley and James started trying to get pregnant after getting married in 2001. "Even though I knew my period was coming, I was compulsive when we first started trying and bought a lot of pregnancy tests," Ashley remembers.. "The tests we did certainly cost hundreds of dollars. We saw making love as labor, which detracted from its delight and satisfaction."

When they finally saw a doctor, they learned that James' sperm count was low. You might be surprised to hear that up to half of all cases of infertility worldwide are caused by male factors, and that up to 2% of individuals with testicles will have poor sperm counts.2.

The couple had to consider the potential that they might not become parents. "I've had days where I didn't want to get out of bed at all."Really, I was down," she says.

Then Ashley experienced a flash of insight. "I simply kept convincing myself that we will become pregnant when the timing was right," she says. "It's hard, and you often think that there's something wrong with you, and there really wasn't."

A few months after accepting that they would not have children, the couple was shocked to learn that they were expecting a kid. Natalie, a daughter, was born in

It All Begins With The Egg:

September of 2003. They were given another surprise years later: the couple didn't even try to conceive the twins.

It Took Ten Months To Become Pregnant.
Amy and Lucas intended to become parents in three months after stopping birth control. "I used to get excited and take a pregnancy test right before my period every month, or I would start my period around testing time. Every month was more depressing than the previous one, according to Amy. "I recall calculating my due date each and every time. Using a phone app, I monitored my temperature and ovulation."

Amy's OB-GYN started her on the fertility medication Clomid after six months. The American College of Obstetricians and Gynecologists (ACOG) advises infertility evaluation and therapy if needed after six months of attempting to conceive for people over 35.3, even though infertility is typically not a worry until a year has elapsed.

Four months ahead of schedule, the Browns scheduled a cruise to commemorate their first anniversary because they felt they deserved a vacation. The month of the cruise was Amy's starting her fourth cycle of Clomid (at an increased dosage). Despite her fatigue prior to the vacation, Amy and Lucas had a great time together, and after returning home, Amy tested positive for pregnancy. She had a baby!

"Our marriage was put to the test by having to wait and be patient, but it also strengthened our bond and increased our gratitude for each other and life itself," the woman says.. July 2011 was when their son was born. Amy thinks it makes sense now that she's thinking back on the trip why she wanted jalapenos on everything!

It Took Fifteen Months To Become Pregnant.
When Melissa and Thomas Murph started attempting to conceive again, they thought the process would be similar to that of getting pregnant with their first daughter, Dakota. "We wanted to have another child, timed so they would be three years apart," Melissa explains. However, she had a negative pregnancy test result each month. She recalls, "I would pray and cry."

It All Begins With The Egg:

The Murphs decided against seeking medical attention and came to terms with the possibility of not having any more children. "At least I have a baby already," I told myself in an attempt to maintain my optimism. According to her, some couples don't even have one.

Melissa realized her period was late and she didn't feel well soon after the pair started accepting what they believed to be their fate. She thought she wasn't pregnant after 14 negative pregnancy tests.

However, she took one more test and eventually received a favorable outcome. Before she was persuaded to tell Thomas the news, she took two additional tests. She says, "We both shed tears." July 2010 saw the birth of Baby Cheyenne.

It Took Five Years To Become Pregnant.
After Dana stopped taking birth control, Chris and Dana had no luck for a year. Following that, they began fertility treatments such as intrauterine insemination (IUI) and Clomid.

The pair continued to take pregnancy tests and try to conceive even when she took pauses from the treatments. "Every time one of my sisters, friends, etc., revealed what she was expecting, it was the lowest moment," remembers Dana.. "During that five-year period, three of my siblings conceived, and my brother's wife actually conceived twice."

Dana found it helpful to keep a notebook. "No one could ever make me feel better when we were trying to conceive," she claims. "It's a demanding process that puts a lot of strain on the partnership."

After almost sixty negative tests, she had a call from God one day from a work acquaintance named Heidi, who was unaware of Dana's situation. It was revealed to her by God that Dana would give birth to a girl.

While taking a break from fertility treatments, the Hernandezes continued to attempt, and two weeks later, Dana's test result was positive. This indicated that

Heidi had made her call two days postpartum. May 2008 saw the birth of Baby Heidi.

It Took Two Years To Become Pregnant.

Tia claims that although she tried for years prior with her former spouse, she and her boyfriend only began trying to conceive in February 2012. "After many misdiagnoses, I was finally told in February of 2014 that I had PCOS (polycystic ovary syndrome)," Tia recounts. She had not ovulated in years and had an extremely high level of estrogen, which makes it difficult for a person to become pregnant.

One of the most frequent reasons for infertility, PCOS affects one in ten persons who are capable of becoming pregnant.5. Luckily, there is treatment for it. Among the methods for addressing infertility brought on by PCOS are:

- *Getting in shape*
- *Drugs (such as Clomid)*
- *IVF (in vitro fertilization) Surgery to start ovulation again*

"We tried everything that could be thought of to help us get pregnant: headstands a lot in our bedroom, acupuncture, chiropractic adjustments, acrobatics, basal temperature monitoring, you name it.! But when Clomid was recommended to us, it completely changed everything! On May 7, I started taking five pills, and on June 8, I got a positive pregnancy test," she recalls.

Tips from Tia for individuals who are having trouble becoming pregnant? Engage in play with one another. Pregnancy struggles are such an emotionally draining journey. Kids, pregnant women, and baby-related stuff are all around you and constantly in your face, the speaker claims. Even though it could feel overwhelming, remember that you have someone who is willing to work with you on this incredibly challenging task.

Talk about it as well; join a support group for fertility or ask for help from someone you can trust. It's crucial to be able to communicate your emotions to people who get you and to accept how hard you're working to accomplish your goals.

It All Begins With The Egg:

"The challenges involved in conception are comparable to those of grieving. Experience your emotions. Have faith in the impossibility. Have faith in your instincts. Get ready for the shift in hormones. Treat yourself well," Tia advises.

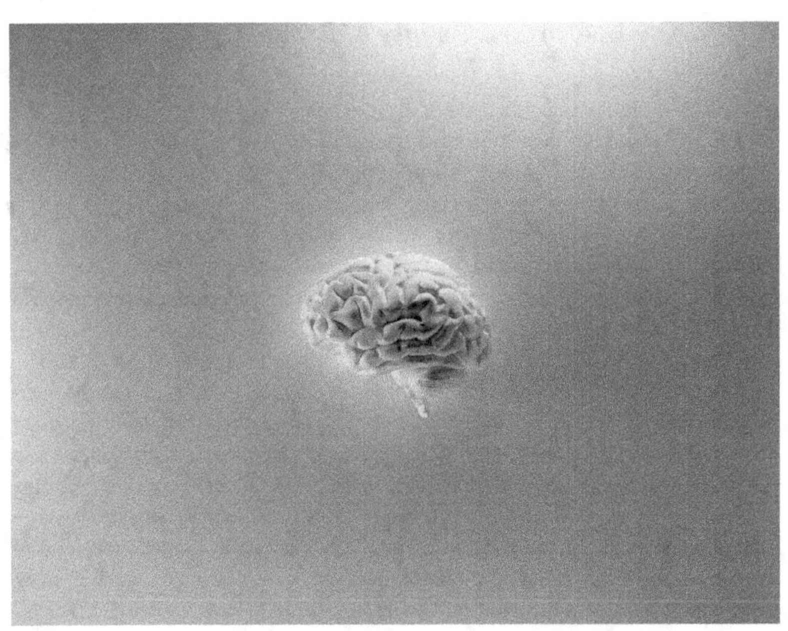

Chapter 7
The Role of Egg Quality in Brain Development

Chapter 7

The Role of Egg Quality in Brain Development

There is a strong body of data backing up the theory that the nutritional status of mothers and children significantly affects the cognitive development of children. Manuscripts from the Industrial Revolution and the Age of Enlightenment, along with ancient texts, emphasize the significance of maternal health and well-being in generating robust, healthy offspring. Furthermore, the quality of the infant's principal nutritional source—breast milk—is directly impacted by the nutritional state and overall health of the postpartum mother. The postnatal diet of the newborn has a significant influence on its cognitive development both during and after birth. Because of how evident these effects were in the past, human milk substitutes were used to care for newborns whose mothers were unable to provide them enough nourishment. Myron Winick and associates' groundbreaking work from the early 1960s provides the foundation for current research on the impact of fetal and neonatal dietary status on cognitive development (Winick and Rosso, 1969). His research showed that brain size, neuronal quantity, and neuronal complexity are all reduced in intrauterine growth restriction (IUGR) caused by starvation. One of the main causes of IUGR worldwide is maternal malnutrition during pregnancy, a potentially preventable illness. Children in societies where moms suffer from chronic malnutrition are also likely to be malnourished. The last trimester of fetal life and the first three years after birth are critical periods for human brain development (Dobbing and Sands, 1979; Thompson and Nelson, 2001). Therefore, it is not surprising that a malnourished mother-fetus/infant dyad poses a significant risk to cognitive development. According to estimates, correcting nutritional deficiencies could increase the global intelligence quotient (IQ) by ten points (Morris, Cogill, and Uauy, 2008).

Essential Nutrients For Developing Babies' Brains

If you've ever spent time with a toddler, you are probably aware of how rapidly they pick up new skills and knowledge. However, a child's brain develops long before they can walk or speak.

A baby's brain grows in the womb at an astounding pace of cell multiplication. Hence, you should place priority on your diet before and during conception.

Motor skills like balance and coordination emerge during infancy, the brain continues to expand. The toddler years (ages 1 to 3) are a time when the brain develops cognitive ability, or the child's capacity to process and apply knowledge rapidly enough to do complicated activities.

Nutrition is crucial during these times of maximum growth. Not giving toddlers the proper nutrition can have a negative effect on their cognitive development, which can subsequently harm their memory, attention, and academic performance.

Essential Nutrients For Developing Babies' Brains

Certain nutrients are more crucial for early brain development than others, even though all nutrients are necessary for brain development and function. The Committee on Nutrition of the American Academy of Pediatrics suggests the following nutrients for toddlers' healthy brain development:

- Iodine
- Choline, and Folate
- Iron
- Long-chain polyunsaturated fatty acids, such as omega-3 fatty acids.
- Zinc
- Protein
- vitamins A, D, B6, and B12

The Best Foods For A Baby's Or Toddler's Developing Brain

There is no one "superfood" or diet that can guarantee toddlers' brain development at its best. However, some meals are rich in many of the essential nutrients. Just watch out for any new foods to make sure there aren't any potential allergies.

1) Eggs

Eggs are a popular choice among young toddlers and are packed with nutrients. Eggs are a good source of protein, vitamin B12, and choline. In particular, choline is critical for healthy brain growth and can enhance cognitive performance. Children ages 8 and under require choline, which can be obtained from two whole eggs per day.

2) Fish

When it comes to brain development, oily fish and other seafood are very beneficial since they contain protein, zinc, iron, choline, iodine, and omega-3 fats. However, steer clear of giving your toddler seafood like swordfish and tuna that is high in mercury. The growing neurological system of a youngster may be negatively impacted by excessive mercury exposure. Rather, choose seafood that is low in mercury, including shrimp, salmon, tilapia, crab, or cod. A 1-ounce portion is permitted for kids under the age of three two or three times a week.

3) Vegetables With Leaves

Parents attempt to conceal additional healthy greens, including kale and spinach, in their kids' smoothies and pasta sauce for a reason: They're an excellent source of folate and iron. Studies reveal that kids who receive adequate folate typically have stronger cognitive abilities than youngsters who don't. The hippocampus, the area of the brain in charge of memory and learning, develops in large part due to iron.

4) Lean Beef Or A Meat Substitute

Because lean beef is a great source of iron and zinc, it is a great brain food. Because young children are more likely to suffer from anemia (low iron levels), iron is very important for them. An iron deficiency affects almost one in ten American children under the age of three, and it can exacerbate learning challenges and attention deficit hyperactivity disorder (ADHD). Soy or black bean burgers are excellent alternatives to burgers that contain iron.

5) Milk

Yogurt without added sugar is a simple, kid-friendly technique to promote brain development. It is packed with minerals, including zinc, choline, protein, and iodine. Thyroid hormones, which are essential for brain development and neurological functions, are produced by children using iodine. The general cognitive function and reasoning skills of a youngster might be impacted by even a modest iodine shortage.

It All Begins With The Egg:

6) Seeds And Nuts

Nuts, seeds, and nut butters are high in zinc and protein and make a great snack. Long-term memory formation and healthy brain growth are facilitated by protein. During the toddler years, when the brain is developing quickly, zinc is also crucial. Your child's cognitive development may be hampered by insufficient zinc, which could impact their memory and learning capacity.

Give peanut-flavored "puff" snacks or dilute small amounts of peanut butter with water to prevent whole nuts and seeds from becoming choking hazards. Just be sure to select puffs that are free of artificial flavors and manufactured from actual peanuts.

7) Lentils

Beans provide zinc, iron, protein, folate, and choline, among other elements that are good for the developing brain. High concentrations of omega-3 fatty acids are also present in some bean varieties, including pinto, kidney, and soybeans. The iron and protein in beans make them a great meat alternative for kids who are vegetarians.

Insights Into Prenatal And Postnatal Care For Optimal Brain Development

What Is Prenatal Care?

Prenatal care refers to the medical attention a woman receives prior to, throughout, and during her pregnancy. Prenatal care must be received on a regular basis by a woman in order to protect her health and the health of her unborn child.

When a woman suspects she is pregnant or does a home pregnancy test to confirm the pregnancy, she should often schedule an appointment with a healthcare professional to start prenatal care. In order to verify the pregnancy and establish the due date, the medical professional will conduct a physical examination and prescribe blood and urine tests.

Throughout prenatal care, the mother's and baby's health will be regularly checked by the healthcare provider, who may also conduct tests, including as blood and ultrasounds, to assess the mother's health and the baby's development. In addition, the healthcare practitioner will counsel and encourage the expectant mother regarding diet, physical activity, and birthing.

Prenatal care must be received on a regular basis by a woman in order to protect her health and the health of her unborn child.

Pregnant women can benefit greatly from physical therapy, which can help both you and your unborn child before, during, and after your pregnancy. The weight of a developing baby can result in posture changes, lower back pain, leg pain, or musculoskeletal problems that were already present before the pregnancy and are now causing pain or discomfort.

Nutrition During Pregnancy
Given that the mother's health and nutrition during her pregnancy can have a substantial impact on the health of the developing baby, prenatal nutrition is an essential component of prenatal care.

A woman's nutritional requirements rise throughout pregnancy in order to support the fetus's growth and development. Pregnant women should eat a varied, balanced diet rich in a variety of nutrients, including fats, proteins, carbs, and vitamins and minerals.

Several Particular Nutrients Are Very Crucial During Pregnancy
1) Folic Acid: Folic acid is a B vitamin that is necessary for the neural tube, which develops into the brain and spinal cord, to grow in the developing fetus. During the first trimester of pregnancy, women should take 400 mcg of folic acid every day.

2) Iron: The synthesis of red blood cells and the delivery of oxygen to the fetus depend on this mineral. To support the increased blood volume during pregnancy, pregnant women require additional iron.

3) Calcium: This mineral is necessary for the growth of a baby's teeth and bones. More calcium is required by pregnant women in order to support the growing baby and preserve the health of their own bones.

Supplements For Pregnancy

To make sure a pregnant woman is getting enough of a certain nutrient, a healthcare professional may occasionally advise using prenatal supplements. Prenatal supplements can include a variety of nutrients, including calcium, iron, and folic acid, and are made especially for expectant mothers. Before beginning any new supplement regimen, it's crucial to talk with a healthcare professional about the usage of prenatal supplements.

Prenatal Care Important For Brain Development

A child's early years have a significant impact on their growth and health later in life. The brain's rapid growth from conception to early childhood is one of the primary causes. Even while the brain changes and develops throughout adulthood, the first eight years of life can lay the groundwork for future learning, good health, and success in life.

A person's brain development is influenced by other variables besides genetics, including:

- appropriate diet beginning with pregnancy

- exposure to pathogens or pollutants

- The child's encounters with the world and other people

The secret to promoting a child's healthy brain development is to provide them with responsive, loving care for both their body and mind. A child's development can be shaped by a combination of positive and unpleasant events that might have a lasting impact. Parents and other caregivers require assistance and the appropriate tools in order to nourish their child's body and mind. Ensuring that children receive the proper care from infancy onwards guarantees that their brains develop normally and attain their maximum potential.

It All Begins With The Egg:

The Significance Of Early Experiences For Brain Development In Children
Children have a lot of talents to learn throughout many years and are ready to learn from birth. Their primary educators are their parents, relatives, and other caregivers, who help them acquire the skills necessary to become self-sufficient and lead successful, healthy lives. A child's experiences with other people and their external surroundings have a big influence on how their brain grows. Mental well-being is essential for brain development. Children develop and learn best in a secure setting with lots of opportunity for play and exploration, shielded from abuse and from severe or ongoing stress.

By talking to, playing with, and taking care of their child, parents and other caregivers can promote healthy brain development in children. When parents build on their child's interests and abilities while taking turns chatting and playing, it helps the child learn most effectively. Children's brains are shielded from stress when their needs are met with understanding and compassion. Children's language and communication skills are strengthened through conversation with adults and exposure to books, stories, and music, setting them up for success in school.

A child's brain may suffer long-term harm from stress and trauma, yet play, reading, and conversation can promote brain development. An essential public health objective is ensuring that parents, caregivers, and early childhood care providers have the tools and knowledge necessary to offer secure, stable, caring, and stimulating care.

Monitoring children's growth and ensuring they meet developmental milestones can assist guarantee that, in cases where children are at risk, any issues are identified early on and that the children receive the necessary intervention.

A Brain's Healthy Beginning
A baby's brain has to be healthy and shielded from illnesses and other hazards in order for it to develop and learn as it should. It is possible to begin fostering a healthy brain's growth even before becoming pregnant. For instance, a balanced diet and the correct nutrients, such as enough folic acid, will support both a healthy pregnancy and a developing baby's neurological system. Immunizations help shield expectant mothers against diseases that could damage the developing brain.

It All Begins With The Egg:

The brain is susceptible to various dangers during pregnancy, including infections like Zika or Cytomegalovirus, exposure to toxins from alcohol or tobacco use, stress, trauma, or mental health issues like depression in expectant women. Premature birth is one issue that can be avoided with regular healthcare during pregnancy and may have an impact on the brain development of the unborn child. Conditions like phenylketonuria (PKU), which have the potential to be harmful to a child's brain, can be identified through newborn screening.

The proper attention and nourishment during infancy are still essential for healthy brain development. Children are particularly susceptible to toxic substances like lead, illnesses, and traumatic head injuries because their developing brains make them more susceptible. Immunizations against childhood diseases, including the measles vaccination, can shield kids from potentially fatal side effects like brain edema. Ensuring that parents and other caregivers have access to secure and healthy settings for their child to play and live can support them in giving more caring care.

What Is Postnatal Care?
The medical attention a woman receives after giving birth is referred to as postnatal care. To protect her health and the health and wellbeing of her newborn, a woman must receive the right postpartum care.

After the baby is born, postnatal care typically starts right away and may entail a hospital stay or a visit to the doctor. In addition to monitoring the mother's and infant's health, the postnatal care provider will offer guidance and instruction on issues like breastfeeding, caring for a newborn, and postpartum recuperation.

The healthcare professional may also answer any worries or inquiries the mother may have regarding the postpartum phase and offer advice on family planning and contraception.

For the sake of the mother's and the newborn's health and wellbeing, it is crucial that a woman have the right postnatal care. This could entail routine check-ups with a medical professional, self-care, and encouragement from loved ones.

Postnatal Care Important For Brain Development
The process of nourishing a child's brain continues into the crucial postnatal care phases after conception. The essential components of postnatal care that support a child's brain development at its best, laying the groundwork for cognitive development, emotional stability, and lifetime learning.

Postnatal care for the best possible development of the brain involves a comprehensive strategy that takes into account the baby's nutritional requirements, emotional ties, cognitive stimulation, sleep hygiene, physical activity, surroundings, and regular medical check-ups. This all-encompassing postnatal care establishes the foundation for a child's development of cognitive abilities, emotional fortitude, and the components of a robust, healthy mind.These care includes:

1) Nutritional Assistance: Energizing Developing Brains
The nutrients received after birth are crucial for brain development. You should seek to breastfeed your child or select suitable formulas that are high in choline, DHA, and omega-3 fatty acids, among other vital nutrients. During the critical early years, these nutrients are essential for myelination, synapse development, and overall cognitive function.

2) Developing Emotional Intelligence through Responsive Care and Bonding
It is critical that infants and caregivers develop close emotional bonds. The importance of providing responsive care, creating safe havens and strong emotional ties, nurturing an atmosphere that offers emotional support is essential for the growth of emotional intelligence and the control of stress reactions of your child.

3. Enhancing Learning Environments through Cognitive Stimulation
Since the brain develops quickly during the perinatal period, cognitive stimulation is crucial. The value of interactive experiences that appeal to the senses, age-appropriate toys, and stimulating activities can not be overemphasized. These stimulating surroundings promote language development, the formation of neural connections, and the learning of cognitive abilities.

4. Sleep Hygiene: How Rest Affects Cognitive Development
Sleeping well is essential for brain growth. Sleeping well is important to develop healthy sleep habits, highlighting how important enough sleep is for memory consolidation, synaptic pruning, and general cognitive performance. Maintaining a regular sleep schedule helps the brain develop as best it can in the postnatal stage.

5. Exercise: Developing Robust Bodies and Minds
Engaging in physical activity not only promotes bodily well-being but also fosters cognitive growth. The relationship between brain function and movement, highlight the value of developmental activities that are appropriate for each child's age and that foster motor skills, coordination, and spatial awareness.

6. Reducing External Stressors: Creating a Calm Environment for Development
The goal of a caring postnatal environment is to reduce stress. The detrimental effects that excessive noise, bright lighting, or chaotic environments can have on a developing brain is overwhelming. Hence, establishing a serene and consistent atmosphere for your child promotes optimal brain growth and psychological welfare.

7) Regular Medical Exams: Tracking Developmental Milestones
In order to track growth milestones throughout the postnatal period, routine healthcare visits are crucial. Developmental evaluations, immunizations, and well-baby checkups guarantee early detection of any possible issues and prompt management for the best possible brain health.

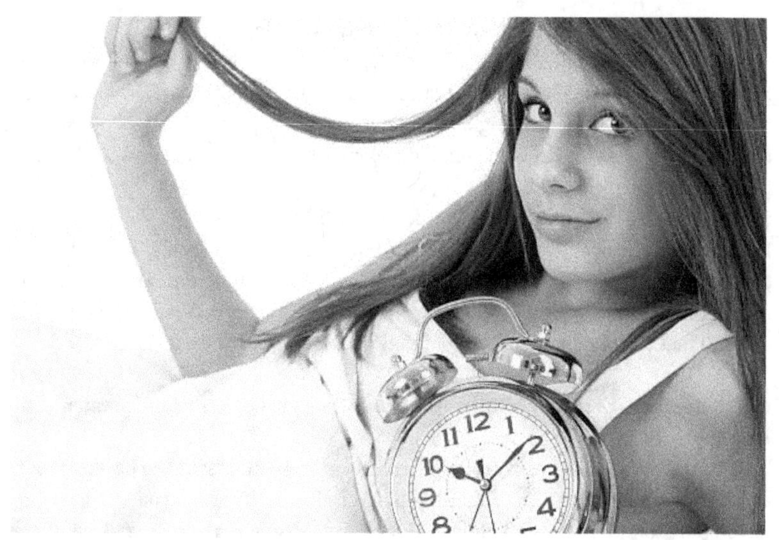

Chapter 8
Fertility Health Across the Lifespan

Chapter 8

Fertility Health Across the Lifespan

Fertility Considerations At Different Stages Of Life

Approximately one to two million immature egg follicles are present in the birth canal of many females. Approximately 400,000 of those eggs are left when menstruation begins, which happens at the age of 12.

Every menstrual cycle, hundreds of eggs are lost. The strongest follicles will develop into mature eggs. The rest is absorbed by the body after breakdown. On the other hand, males spend the majority of their adult life producing new sperm.

The body loses follicles as it ages. As a result, the follicles have less chances to produce robust, healthy eggs for fertilization. Although there is a plentiful supply during adolescence, by the late 30s and early 40s, it is beginning to diminish. Still, an increasing number of people are trying to start families at that age.

According to a reliable source, the average age of a first-time mother nowadays is 26. years old. Due to the delay of parenthood, that age has been rising gradually in recent years.

Let's Examine How Delaying Can Impact Your Ability To Conceive.

i) 18 To 24 Years Of Age
If there was ever an "optimal" age to have children solely based on physical attributes, this would be it.

Your younger eggs are more likely to be of a higher caliber since your body's strongest ovarian follicles grow into eggs before they are ready for ovulation.

Having a child at this age will reduce the chance of:

- birth defects

- Chromosome issues

- a few problems with fertility

- Of course, having children between the ages of 18 and 24 is not without risk, even though it is less risky.

Your fecundity rate, or likelihood of being fertile, will fluctuate throughout your life. It is at its peak during this younger stage of life. The monthly natural fertility rate between the ages of 20 and 30 is approximately 25%. After 35, that decreases to less than 10%.

For females aged 18 to 24, the birth rate is declining. Up until their 30s and 40s, many people choose to put their professions ahead of their families.

ii) 25 To 30 Years Old
Your chances of getting pregnant naturally decrease with each year that goes by. However, your likelihood of becoming pregnant on your own in your late 20s is quite constant.

According to estimates from the Eunice Kennedy Shriver National Institute of Child Health and Human Development, couples under 30 who are otherwise healthy can conceive 40 to 60 percent of the time in their first three months of trying. The likelihood of becoming pregnant declines annually beyond the age of thirty.

Don't panic if you haven't yet started a family! When the time is appropriate, your body will still produce an abundance of eggs.

However, consult your doctor if you've been trying to conceive for at least three months and are still having trouble. Even though the majority of couples at this age can conceive naturally, some advice might be useful.

iii) 31 To 35 Years Old

You still have a good possibility of becoming pregnant in your early 30s.

At this age, your odds will start to steadily fall, but you still have a lot of quality eggs to offer. Up until the age of 32, your fecundity rate gradually declines. After 37, it sharply declines. You are around half as fertile in your 30s as you were in your early 20s.

Does that imply that if you're in your 30s, you can't be a parent? Not at all.

According to the National Institutes of Health, 1 in 5 women in the country give birth to their first child after the age of 35. On the other hand, one in three couples in their 30s will struggle with infertility.

iv) 35 And 40 Years Old

The late 30s and early 40s see the biggest decline in fertility. A woman in her late 30s has roughly half the probability of conceiving naturally compared to a woman in her early 20s.

An analysis from 2003 According to Trusted Source, 85% of couples in this age group will be able to conceive within two years, while 60% of them will be able to conceive naturally within a year of beginning to try.

Nonetheless, there is a greater chance of chromosomal problems with eggs at this age. The risks rise with each passing year. This implies that there is a greater chance of miscarriage or unplanned pregnancy.

The decade of life in which more people than ever are attempting to become pregnant also happens to correspond with this decline in fertility rates.

According to data from the Centers for Disease Control and Prevention (CDC), the birth rate for females aged 35 to 39 increased annually from 2011 to 2016, but it decreased by 1% in 2017. The birth rate is substantially greater for females over 39.

41 To 45 Years Old And Older

The CDC reports that between 2016 and 2017, the birth rate for people aged 40 to 44 rose by 2%. During the same period, there was a 3% increase in the number of births among females aged 45 to 49. In actuality, women 40 years of age and above have the fastest-growing rates of childbearing.

Though more people are giving birth at these ages, the overall percentage of births to older parents is still far lower than that of younger ones, so it's crucial to keep that in mind. This is partly because getting pregnant after 40 is more difficult.

Your body is getting ready for menopause at this age. It's likely that your ovaries have used up all of their follicles or are almost out. With every cycle that goes by, more will vanish. You won't have many follicles left by the time you're in your early 50s'

Additionally, there is an increased chance of various birth abnormalities and pregnancy difficulties for babies born to individuals in this age group. This stage of life is marked by a high increase in chromosomal abnormalities and miscarriages.

Additionally, becoming older raises the parent's chance of issues such as:

- Hypertension

- Diabetes

- preeclampsia

People are delaying starting families longer these days. Due to developments in reproductive therapies, like in vitro fertilization, these people frequently become pregnant at this later stage.

Fertility therapies may be able to prolong your window and perhaps increase your chances of a successful conception, even if your natural window usually closes as you age.

The Age And Fertility Of Men

Although it has long been known that a woman's age impacts her fertility, more recent research has revealed that a man's age also influences a woman's chances of becoming pregnant and the health of her unborn child.

When Sperm Quality Declines: male fertility often begins to decline between the ages of 40 and 45. Male age increases are associated with a decrease in the likelihood of conception overall, an increase in the time to conception (the number of menstrual cycles required to become pregnant), and a higher risk of miscarriage and fetal mortality.

The likelihood of mental health issues in children of older fathers is also higher (but still uncommon). Compared to children whose fathers are 30 years of age or younger, children whose fathers are 40 or older are five times more likely to suffer from autism spectrum disorder. Additionally, they have a somewhat higher chance of experiencing schizophrenia and other mental health issues in the future.

Age-Related Fertility Challenges And Solutions

Age has an increasingly important role in determining reproductive patterns as people get older. Comprehending the obstacles linked to the age-related decrease in fertility and investigating workable remedies are essential measures for individuals managing family planning at various phases.

Resolving age-related fertility issues calls for a diverse strategy that includes everything from proactive family planning and understanding biological timeframes to utilizing assisted reproductive technology and placing a high priority on general health and wellness. Through the use of knowledge, proactive thinking, and help in overcoming these obstacles, individuals and couples can make decisions that are in line with their particular reproductive path.

The intricacies, factors, and possible remedies for age-related reproduction problems are listed below:

1) The Biological Clock: Comprehending Fertility Decline Associated with Age

The amount and quality of eggs naturally decline with aging in women. Fertility is impacted by the reduction in ovarian reserve and the elevated risk of chromosomal abnormalities. Men's reproductive systems may continue to function as they age, but the quality of their sperm may decline. Comprehending this biological clock is essential to tackling age-related reproductive issues.

2) Obstacles to Female Fertility: Reducing Ovarian Reserve and Raising Risks

A woman's declining ovarian reserve may make it more difficult for her to conceive, prolong the time it takes to get pregnant, and raise her chance of miscarriage. Proactive family planning, taking into account assisted reproductive technologies (ART) such as in vitro fertilization (IVF), and being cognizant of the possibility of needing fertility treatments as one ages are some of the solutions.

3) Issues with Male Fertility: Aging Sperm and Sperm Quality

Men can generate sperm for the rest of their lives, but the quality of their sperm may decline with age. This may have an impact on reproductive results and raise the possibility of genetic disorders in progeny. A healthy lifestyle, taking care of any potential health problems, and getting prompt fertility tests are some of the solutions.

4) Actively Organizing Your Family: Handling the Biological Schedule

Knowing how age affects fertility highlights the significance of early family planning. In order to maintain their potential for fertility, women are advised to think about their reproductive aspirations early on and look into methods like egg freezing. Navigating the intricacies of family planning timeframes requires open communication and collaborative decision-making among partners.

5) Closing the Distance with Assisted Reproductive Technologies (ART)

ART shows promise as a treatment for individuals with age-related infertility issues. Technologies that can increase the likelihood of conception include preimplantation genetic testing (PGT), intracytoplasmic sperm injection (ICSI), and in vitro fertilization (IVF). Success rates can differ, though, and a number of variables—including general health—are important.

It All Begins With The Egg:

6) Lifestyle and Well-Being: Enhancing Health of Fertility
At any age, it is critical to optimize fertility health through lifestyle decisions. Reproductive health is enhanced by eating a balanced diet, getting regular exercise, controlling stress, and abstaining from dangerous substances. These behaviors can somewhat reduce age-related difficulties and have a good effect on fertility.

7) Empowering Individuals and Couples via Education and Support
Support groups and educational programs are essential for enabling individuals and couples to make knowledgeable decisions regarding their reproductive journey. Having access to trustworthy information, therapy, and emotional support can assist manage the psychological effects of age-related fertility difficulties.

CONCLUSION

And that, my dear readers, concludes our fertility fiesta. We've negotiated the twists and turns of egg quality, danced through the complexities of conception, and even had a few laughs in the process. As we say goodbye, I'd like to leave you with a shot of knowledge, a sprinkling of humor, and a whole lot of optimism.

Remember that fertility is a journey, not a sprint. Your story, like a fascinating thriller, may include surprising plot twists, triumphant moments, and perhaps a tearjerker or two. But here's a secret: you are the author of your fertility story, and you write every chapter.

In our investigation into the science of egg quality, we discovered the value of knowledge. Armed with this knowledge, you are no longer just a passenger on this reproductive rollercoaster; you are the one driving it. Whether you're exploring assisted reproductive technologies, natural conception tactics, or simply enjoying the ride, know that you have the resources to make informed decisions.

Now, as you close the book and begin your own reproductive journey, remember the lessons, laughter, and perseverance we shared. Life is unpredictable, as is the mystery of generating life. Accept the uncertainty, cherish the wins, and keep your sense of humor nearby - you'll need it!

I am grateful to each and every reader who joined me on this voyage. Your tales, hardships, and victories have made this trip more fulfilling than I could have dreamed. Remember, you are not alone on this journey, and the network of fertility fighters is large and strong.

As you embark on the next chapter of your life, may it be filled with the pitter-patter of small feet, the joy of starting a family, and a sense of accomplishment that transcends the pages of this book. Here's to new beginnings, productive journeys, and great stories still to be told.

I wish you all the joy, love, and luck on your individual fertility journey. Until we meet again, remain safe, optimistic, and keep the eggcellent spirit alive!

It All Begins With The Egg:

With thanks and kindest wishes,
Teresa J. Macek ✸ ⬤ ✦